Zsolt Radak (ed.)

Exercise and Diseases

Prevention through Training

Meyer & Meyer Sport

British Library Cataloguing in Publication Data
A catalogue record for this book is available from the British Library

Zsolt Radak (ed.)
Exercise and Diseases: Prevention through Training
– Oxford: Meyer & Meyer Sport (UK) Ltd., 2005
ISBN 1-84126-121-1

© 2005 by Meyer & Meyer Sport (UK) Ltd.
Aachen, Adelaide, Auckland, Budapest, Graz, Johannesburg,
New York, Olten (CH), Oxford, Singapore, Toronto
Member of the World
Sports Publishers' Association
www.w-s-p-a.org

Printed and bound in Germany by: Mennicken, Aachen
ISBN 1-84126-121-1
E-Mail: verlag@m-m-sports.com
www.m-m-sports.com

Contents

Exercise and Type 2 Diabetes Mellitus

Exercise and Cancer

Alzheimer as a Disease of Metabolic Demand: Benefits of Physical and Brain Exercise

GEORGE PERRY[1], ROBERT P. FRIEDLAND[2], GRACE J. PETOT[3], AKIHIKO NUNOMURA[4],
RUDOLPH J. CASTELLANI[1,5], ZVEZDANA KUBAT[1] AND MARK A. SMITH[1]

[1]Institute of Pathology
[2]Department of Neurology
[3]Department of Nutrition, Case Western Reserve University, Cleveland, Ohio 44106 USA
[4]Department of Psychiatry and Neurology, Asahikawa Medical College, Asahikawa 078-8510, Japan
[5]Department of Pathology, Michigan State University, East Lansing, Michigan 48824, USA

Correspondence to:

George Perry, Ph.D.
Institute of Pathology
Case Western Reserve University
2085 Adelbert Road
Cleveland, Ohio 44106 USA
216-368-2488
216-368-8964 (fax)
george.perry@case.edu

Summary

A growing body of evidence suggests that the deficits of Alzheimer disease stem from metabolic deficits. These metabolic deficits may play a role in initiating the pathological changes that have been the major focus of study. Intervention to remedy the metabolic deficits may prevent or lessen the development of Alzheimer disease. Consistent with this view, metabolic conditioning, through physical or mental exercise, reduces the incidence of Alzheimer disease and leads us to consider that therapeutic strategies focused on metabolic enhancement and exercise as well as agents that assist these processes may benefit patients.

Introduction

The age-related increase in the incidence of Alzheimer disease (AD) is one of the most striking features of this condition and, arguably, the most important. In those lacking autosomal dominant inheritance, prior to 60 years of age, AD is almost non-existent, whereas by the age of 85, nearly half of the population suffers from AD (Perry and Smith, 1999). While pathological loss of cognitive function increases with aging for the majority of individuals, functional cognition is maintained even though other abilities, such as muscle strength and endurance, are greatly reduced. The defining feature of *Homo sapiens* is higher cognition, which separates us from all other organisms by orders of magnitude even though we are genetically separated by only one percent from our closest relative. Therefore, while function of the brain and heart has priority for all organisms to maintain life, it is function of the former, requiring 20-25% of basal metabolism, which defines humanity. In this article, we review recent evidence indicating that retention of cognitive function during aging may be brought about by metabolic alterations that can be modified by mental and/or physical exercise.

Oxidative Imbalance and Mitochondrial Abnormalities in Alzheimer Disease

While the brain-body connection has been evident for millennia, its role in AD is only becoming apparent. Almost twenty years ago, cell culture studies showed metabolic deficits in non-neuronal cells from AD patients and recent studies point to mitochondrial abnormalities in such cells (Ghosh et al., 1999; Trimmer et al., 2000). These findings further suggest that AD, generally considered a brain disorder, may involve other tissue types.

In our own studies of oxidative balance in AD, we have focused our efforts on the major site of damage - the cell bodies of neurons involved in AD. These large, highly metabolic cells show extensive damage to every category of macromolecule: lipid (Sayre et al., 1997), protein (Smith et al., 1996), sugar (Smith et al., 1994) and nucleic acid (Nunomura et al., 1999). Damage is pronounced and apparent early in the course of AD, probably predating cognitive deficits. That oxidative damage is early is based on quantitative assessment of oxidative damage showing levels are highest in newly diagnosed cases and decreases with disease duration (Nunomura et al., 2001). Further, in Down syndrome where amyloid deposition can be detected at about 25 years of age, oxidative damage increases more than a decade earlier (Nunomura et al., 2000).

Oxidative imbalance is likely precipated by an accumulation of mitochondrial (mtDNA) in all vulnerable neurons where ultrastructural analysis shows the accumulated mtDNA restricted to lipofuscin-associated lysosomes, the remnants of autophagy. Morphometrically, there is a small, but significant, decrease in mitochondria in AD. These findings suggest that profound changes in mitochondria dynamics occur early in the course of AD (Ghosh et al., 1999). The increased remnants of autophagy indicate that neuron specificity might be related to reduction of organelle transport, as first suggested by Terry (Suzuki and Terry, 1967; Terry, 2000). The mitochondria remnants we find in AD are likely the consequence of mitochondrial retention and turnover in the cell body due to reduced export to the axon. Consistent with this interpretation, we found a profound reduction of microtubules, the conduit of mitochondria, in neurons in AD, even when neurofibrillary tangles were absent (Cash et al., 2003). The reason why mitochondrial autophagy and the full spectrum of oxidative damage is restricted to vulnerable neurons and not seen in other cell types is unclear. It may be that different cell types have the same fundamental deficit, but expression is highly dependent on physiology, e.g., energy requirements, transport properties and the importance of antioxidant defenses.

Some of the major proteins involved in AD pathology, amyloid protein precursor, presenilin 1, and secretase (BACE), have been localized to cells of the pancreas (Figueroa et al., 2001), the site of insulin production. This opens the possibility that reduced cerebral glucose utilization prior to dementia (Small et al., 1996) reflects a fundamental abnormality in brain glucose metabolism. Further, the finding that vascular atrophy correlates with the extent of amyloid deposits could reflect disuse atrophy of vessels through lower demand, rather than vascular-driven amyloid deposition (de la Torre, 1996; Perry et al., 1998).

Benefits of Physical Exercise

If AD reflects reduced metabolic capacity with aging, could use and conditioning, i.e., exercise, be of benefit? In a case control study of physical exercise, we found a protective effect from AD (Friedland et al., 2000). Responses to a life-history questionnaire of physical exercise were obtained from 126 subjects with AD, 55 men and 71 women, with a mean age of 77 years (SD = 8.6) and 315 control subjects consisted of 121 men and 194 women, with a mean age of 75 years (SD = 6.1). A physical activity scaled scoring system based on energy expenditure and frequency was used to evaluate each activity. The mean of physical activity values for AD cases was 1.16 (SD = 0.81), and the corresponding value for the controls was 1.44 (SD = 0.60). The mean difference is 0.273 (p < 0.001). AD cases represent a disproportionately large percentage of the group that exercised less, and control cases a disproportionate large percentage of those that exercised more over the 39-year period of analysis. The difference remained statistically significant after controlling for covariates year of birth, gender and education (Friedland et al., 2000).

It is not possible to determine if the association of AD with reduced pre-morbid activities represents a risk factor, an early manifestation of the disease itself, or both. One possible explanation for the benefits of exercise in regard to the development of AD is that neuronal activation, associated with functional activity, spares the brain from the disease process through beneficial effects on membranes and amyloid production, degradation and aggregation.

Mental Activity

One strategy to study the effect of brain activity on onset and progression of AD uses educational attainment as *a priori* evidence of brain activity level. According to this hypothesis, individuals with higher educational attainment engage in a greater degree of mental activity, perhaps at critical periods during cognitive development, and therefore differ, in a positive way, from those less educated in terms of metabolic processes necessary to preserve cognitive function as brain tissue is lost. Evidence of such a process was given by Zhang et al. (1990), who found low education as a highly significant and independent risk factor for dementia in a large Chinese population. They suggested that the possible effects of early deprivation, or lower brain "reserve", may unmask AD early in the disease in those less educated. Similarly, Stern et al. (1994, 1995) found an increase risk of mortality in AD patients with more advanced educational and occupational attainment. They note that while this may at first seem counterintuitive, it implies that at any level of assessed clinical severity, the underlying AD pathology is more advanced in those with more education, resulting in shorter duration of diagnosed disease before death. These data suggest that education may provide a reserve against clinical manifestations early in the course of AD, and decrease the ease of clinical detection. On the other hand, Cobb et al. (1995) found low educational attainment to be a risk factor for dementia also resulting from causes other than AD, suggesting that smoking and other risk factors for atherogenesis and stroke common to lower socioeconomic groups, may underlie the relationship. Additionally, Geerlings et al. (1997) were unable to find a correlation between increased risk of death and educational attainment in AD, while Letenneur et al. (2000) found an association of education with Alzheimer disease in women only. These studies suggest that high levels of cerebral exertion during life may protect against AD.

Apolipoprotein E

Apolipoprotein E genetoype, the major genetic risk factor for AD, is involved in lipid transport. Notably, genetic variation in response to dietary intake has been shown for a number of age-related diseases. We examined dietary factors in a case-control study to investigate the effects of dietary fat intake on the risk of AD associated with the apolipoprotein E 4 allele (Petot et al., 2000). Food frequencies were converted to daily consumption of nutrients. Apolipoprotein E genotype was determined for 72 cases of AD and 232 controls with dietary information from one or more age periods. Apolipoprotein E genotype was dichotomized as those having a 4 allele versus no 4 allele. Modification of risk by dietary fat was determined by stratified analysis and logistic regression controlling for year of birth and education.

The risk for AD, associated with the 4 allele, increased sharply with higher fat intake among both men and women, especially before age 60. For carriers of 4, the risk for AD was over 7 times higher for those with a high fat diet compared to those with a low fat diet. These findings indicate that lower fat diets during early adulthood and midlife may substantially reduce risk of AD, especially for those with an apolipoprotein 4 allele.

While increased lipid peroxidation, as suggested by Montine and Poirier, could be responsible for the effect of 4 allele (Montine et al., 1996; Ramassamy et al., 1999, 2000), we found a more complex relationship (Figure 1). Essentially similar levels of oxidative damage are found in apolipoprotein 4 allele carriers and non-carriers, yet only apolipoprotein 4 allele carriers showed a relationship to amyloid deposits. These findings suggest that apolipoprotein 4 is linked to the relationship of oxidative damage and amyloid. Moreover, this may indicate that apolipoprotein 4 allele carriers require greater amyloid antioxidant activity (Cuajungco et al., 2000).

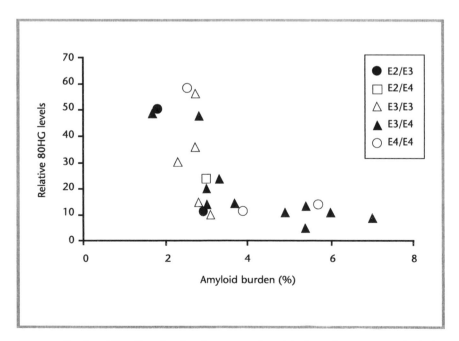

Figure 1. In AD, the level of neuronal oxidative damage marked by 8-hydroxyguanosine (8OHG) is inversely related to amyloid B deposition, most strikingly for cases carrying at least one copy of the apolipoprotein E 4 allele.

Changes Begin with Aging

We have found that metabolic imbalance is apparent, in the form of ostensibly benign changes years before the development of AD, likely representing the compensatory mechanisms of the body. Mitochondrial remnants in lysosomes, oxidative damage, and antioxidant responses can be found in most individuals over the age of 40 years, but only at approximately 10-20% of the levels seen in AD. Most striking is that oxidative damage in controls is strongly related to the extent of mitochondrial abnormalities (r^2 = 0.872, p = 0.011) while in AD, oxidative damage is unrelated to the extent of mitochondrial autophagy (r^2 = 0.147) (Figure 2) and is instead related (inversely) (Figure 1) to amyloid deposition and duration of dementia. These distinct relationships seem to mark a phase shift, related to increased demands for antioxidant defenses, and also related to induction of the pentose phosphate pathway (Martins et al., 1986; Russell et al., 1999) and the pleotrophic effect of rerouting priority from energy metabolism (normal neuronal function) to antioxidant defenses (survival), the consequence of which is reduced function.

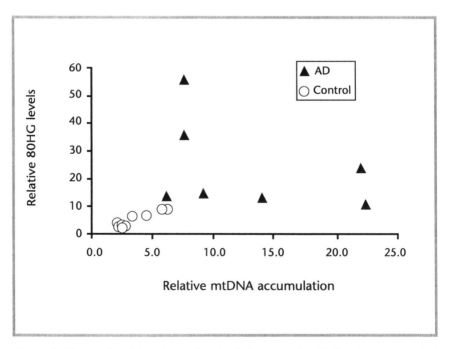

Figure 2. *The relationship between the level of neuronal oxidative damage marked by 8-hydroxyguanosine (8OHG) and mtDNA accumulation is linear for aged controls but more complex for cases with AD.*

Conclusion

When age-related metabolic deficits confront the essential high-energy demands of the human brain, a substantial re-routing of metabolic priority is required to maintain function. Extrinsic parameters, such as good nutrition and exercise, combined with intrinsic factors, such as genetics, offers a unique experience to each individual in their lifetime. The extrinsic factors are those that can be ultimately controlled by the individual and thus exercise and good nutrition during one's lifetime can promote effective energy utilization.

REFERENCES

Cash, A. D., Aliev, G., Siedlak, S. L., Nunomura, A., Fujioka, H., Zhu, X., Raina, A. K., Vinters, H. V., Tabaton, M., Johnson, A. B., Paula-Barbosa, M., Avila, J., Jones, P. K., Castellani, R. J., Smith, M. A., Perry, G. (2003). Microtubule reduction in Alzheimer's disease and aging is independent of tau filament formation. *American Journal of Pathology* 162:1623-1627.

Cobb, J. L., Wolf, P. A, Au, R., White, R., D'Agostino, R. B. (1995). The effect of education on the incidence of dementia and Alzheimer's disease in the Framingham Study. *Neurology* 45:1707-1712.

Cuajungco, M. P., Goldstein, L. E., Nunomura, A., Smith, M. A., Lim, J. T., Atwood, C. S., Huang, X., Farrag, Y. W., Perry, G., Bush, A. I. (2000). Evidence that the ß-amyloid plaques of Alzheimer's disease represent the redox-silencing and entombment of Aß by zinc. *Journal of Biological Chemistry* 275:19439-19442.

de la Torre, J. C. (1999). Critical threshold cerebral hypoperfusion causes Alzheimer's disease? *Acta Neuropathologica* 98:1-8.

Figueroa, D. J., Shi, X.-P., Gardell, S. J., Austin, C. P. (2001). AßPP secretases are co-expressed with AßPP in the pancreatic islets. *Journal of Alzheimer's Disease* 3: 393-396.

Friedland, R. P., Fritsch, T., Smyth, K. A., Koss, E., Lerner, A.J ., Chen, C. H., Petot, G. J., Debanne, S. H. (2000). Intellectual and physical activities are protective against the development of Alzheimer's disease. *Neurobiology of Aging* 21(Suppl 1S):S99.

Geerlings, M.I., Deeg, D.J., Schmand, B., Lindeboom, J., Jonker, C. (1997). Increased risk of mortality in Alzheimer's disease patients with higher education? A replication study. *Neurology* 49:798-802.

Ghosh, S.S., Swerdlow, R.H., Miller, S.W., Sheeman, B., Parker, W.D. Jr., Davis, R.E. (1999). Use of cytoplasmic hybrid cell lines for elucidating the role of mitochondrial dysfunction in Alzheimer's disease and Parkinson's disease. *Annals of the New York Academy of Sciences* 893:176-191.

Letenneur, L., Launer, L. J., Andersen, K., Dewey, M. E., Ott, A., Copeland, J.R., Dartigues, J.F., Kragh-Sorensen, P., Baldereschi, M., Brayne, C., Lobo, A., Martinez-Lage, J.M., Stijnen, T., Hofman, A. (2000). Education and the risk for Alzheimer's disease: sex makes a difference. EURODEM pooled analyses. EURODEM Incidence Research Group. *American Journal of Epidemiology* 151:1064-1071.

Martins, R. N., Harper, C. G., Stokes, G. B., Masters, C. L. (1986). Increased cerebral glucose-6-phosphate dehydrogenase activity in Alzheimer's disease may reflect oxidative stress. *Journal of Neurochemistry* 46:1042-1045.

Montine, T. J., Amarnath, V., Martin, M. E., Strittmatter, W. J., Graham, D. G. (1996). E-4-hydroxy-2-nonenal is cytotoxic and cross-links cytoskeletal proteins in P19 neuroglial cultures. *American Journal of Pathology* 148:89-93.

Nunomura, A., Perry, G., Pappolla, M. A., Wade, R., Hirai, K., Chiba, S., Smith, M.A. (1999) RNA oxidation is a prominent feature of vulnerable neurons in Alzheimer's disease. *Journal of Neuroscience* 19:1959-1964.

Nunomura, A., Perry, G., Hirai, K., Chiba, S., Smith, M. A. (2000). Neuronal oxidative stress precedes amyloid-ß deposition in Down's syndrome. *Journal of Neuropathology and Experimental Neurology* 59:1011-1017.

Nunomura, A., Perry, G., Aliev, G., Hirai, K., Takeda, A., Balraj, E. K., Jones, P. K., Ghanbari, H., Wataya, T., Shimohama, S., Chiba, S., Atwood, C. S., Petersen, R. B., Smith, M. A. (2001). Oxidative damage is the earliest event in Alzheimer disease. *Journal of Neuropathology and Experimental Neurology* 60:759-767.

Perry, G., Smith, M.A., McCann, C.E., Siedlak, S.L., Jones, P.K., Friedland, R.P. (1998). Cerebrovascular muscle atrophy is a feature of Alzheimer's disease. *Brain Research* 791:63-66.

Perry, G., Smith, M.A. (1999). Alzheimer disease. In: *Encyclopedia of Neuroscience*, 2nd Edition, Adelman G, Smith BH, Eds, Elsevier Science BV, Amsterdam, 1999, pp 59-61.

Petot, G.J., Cook, T.B., Riedal, R.M., Chen, C.H., Debanne, S.M., Koss, E., Lerner, A.J., Friedland, R.P. (2000). A high fat diet during adulthood increases risk for Alzheimer's disease for those with the ApoE _4 allele. *Neurobiology of Aging* 21(Suppl 1S):S246.

Ramassamy, C., Averill, D., Beffert, U., Bastianetto, S., Theroux, L., Lussier-Cacan, S., Cohn, J. S., Christen, Y., Davignon, J., Quirion, R., Poirier, J. (1999). Oxidative damage and protection by antioxidants in the frontal cortex of Alzheimer's disease is related to the apolipoprotein E genotype. *Free Radical Biology and Medicine* 27:544-553.

Ramassamy, C., Averill, D., Beffert, U., Theroux, L., Lussier-Cacan, S., Cohn, J. S., Christen, Y., Schoofs, A., Davignon, J., Poirier, J. (2000). Oxidative insults are associated with apolipoprotein E genotype in Alzheimer's disease brain. *Neurobiology of disease* 7:23-37.

Russell, R. L., Siedlak, S. L., Raina, A. K., Bautista, J. M., Smith, M. A., Perry, G. (1999). Increased neuronal glucose-6-phosphate dehydrogenase and sulfhydryl levels indicate reductive compensation to oxidative stress in Alzheimer disease. *Archives of Biochemistry and Biophysics* 370:236-239.

Sayre, L. M., Zelasko, D. A., Harris, P. L. R., Perry, G., Salomon, R. G., Smith, M. A. (1997). 4-Hydroxynonenal-derived advanced lipid peroxidation end products are increased in Alzheimer's disease. *Journal of Neurochemistry* 68:2092-2097.

Small, G.W., Komo, S., La Rue, A., Saxena, S., Phelps, M.E., Mazziotta, J.C., Saunders, A.M., Haines, J.L., Pericak-Vance, M.A., Roses, A.D. (1996). Early detection of Alzheimer's disease by combining apolipoprotein E and neuroimaging. *Annals of the New York Academy of Sciences* 802:70-78.

Smith, M.A., Perry, G., Richey, P.L., Sayre, L.M., Anderson, V.E., Beal, M.F., Kowall, N. (1996). Oxidative damage in Alzheimer's. *Nature* 382:120-121.

Smith, M.A., Taneda, S., Richey, P.L., Miyata, S., Yan, S.-D., Stern, D., Sayre, L.M., Monnier, V.M., Perry, G. (1994). Advanced Maillard reaction end products are associated with Alzheimer disease pathology. *Proceedings of the National Academy of Sciences of the United States of America* 91:5710-5714.

Stern, Y. Gurland, B., Tatemichi, T.K., Tang, M.X., Wilder, D., Mayeux, R. (1994). Influence of education and occupation on the incidence of Alzheimer's disease. *Journal of the American Medical Association* 271:1004-1010.

Stern, Y., Tang, M.X., Denaro, J., Mayeux, R. (1995). Increased risk of mortality in Alzheimer's disease patients with more advanced educational and occupational attainment. *Annals of Neurology* 37:590-595.

Suzuki, K., Terry, R.D. (1967). Fine structural localization of acid phosphatase in senile plaques in Alzheimer's presenile dementia. *Acta Neuropathologica* 8:276-284.

Terry, R.D. (2000). Cell death or synaptic loss in Alzheimer disease. *Journal of Neuropathology and Experimental Neurology* 59:1118-1119.

Trimmer, P. A., Swerdlow, R.H., Parks, J.K., Keeney, P., Bennett, J.P. Jr., Miller, S.W., Davis, R.E., Parker, W.D. Jr. (2000). Abnormal mitochondrial morphology in sporadic Parkinson's and Alzheimer's disease cybrid cell lines. *Experimental Neurology* 162:37-50.

Zhang, M. Y., Katzman, R., Salmon, D., Jin, H., Cai, G. J., Wang, Z. Y., Qu, G. Y., Grant, I., Yu, E., Levy, P., et al. (1990). The prevalence of dementia in Alzheimer's disease in Shanghai, China: impact of age, gender, and education. *Annals of Neurology* 27:428-437.

Exercise and Inflammatory Disease: Beneficial Effects of Exercise as a Stimulus of Hormesis

Hae Young Chung[*1], Hyun Jeen Kim[1], Young Ho Baek[1], Seung Heyg Song[1] and Zsolt Radak[2]

[1] College of Pharmacy/Aging Tissue Bank, Busan National University, Gumjung-Ku, Busan 609-735, Korea.
[2] Faculty of Sport Science, Semmelweis University, Budapest, Hungary

*Correspondence to:

Hae Young Chung, Ph.D.
College of Pharmacy/Aging Tissue Bank
Busan National University
Gumjung-Ku, Busan 609-735
Te/Fax : 82-51-510-2814
e-mail : hyjung@pusan.ac.kr

Summary

The beneficial effects of exercise are interpreted by the hormetic mechanism suggesting that a change in redox state of tissue may act as signal for adaptation. In addition, beneficial effects of nitric oxide (NO) were discussed on both hemodynamic control and metabolic regulation during exercise.

The maintenance of homeostasis in organisms may be due to diverse adaptations to enviromental stress based on a hormesis-type mechanism, which allows low or moderate levels of stimulus such as exercise to stimulate the production of physiological levels of NO and reactive oxygen species.

Introduction

Exercise has been recognized as beneficial in certain contexts but as detrimental when forced for long durations, or when extreme regimens are employed. The immune system is enhanced during mild and moderate exercise (Jonsdottir 2000). However, excessive long-duration exercise is followed by reduced lymphocyte concentration, suppressed non-MHC-restricted cytotoxicity and decreased IgA in mucosa (Juto et al., 1985). The level of immune suppression depends on the intensity and duration of the exercise. Animal studies have shown that regular moderate physical exercise enhances resting level of natural immunity (Jonsdottir et al., 2000).

Excessive physical exercise has been shown to induce an acute response of the immune system, including the activation of inflammatory cells (Nieman,

1997). Metabolic activation correlates with an augmented generation of reactive oxygen species (ROS) and reactive nitrogen species (RNS) by leukocytes, a mechanism that is partly mediated by cytokines such as plasma interleukin-8 (IL-8) and tumor necrosis factor-α (TNF-α) (Cannon, 1990) Protection and/or tolerance against exercise-induced oxidative, heat, cytokine, and inflammatory stress in leukocytes may be in part provided by heat shock proteins (HSPs), antioxidant enzymes, and metallothioneins (Fehrenbach, 1999). The metabolic changes caused by exercise are similar to those known to induce stress protein synthesis and antioxidant enzymes (Flanagan et al., 1990). HSPs play a role in protein translocation, stabilization, assembly, and degradation processes, the functions that could be important in leukocytes activated by excessive exercise (Kaufmann,1990). Metallothionein and antioxidant enzymes also can scavenge ROS to protect cells against oxidative stress.

Inflammation is fundamentally a protective response, the ultimate goal of which is to rid the organism of both the initial causes of cell damage, such as microbes and toxins, and consequences of such injury (e.g. necrotic cells and tissue) (Lapenna et al., 1994). Without inflammation, infections might go unchecked, wounds would never heal and damaged tissue can remain permanent festering sores. However, prolonged, chronic inflammatory reactions, which are uncontrolled by sustained stimuli, may be potentially harmful and life-threatening because of the overproduction of toxic by-products such as ROS and RNS (Lapenna et al., 1994). Representative inflammatory diseases include rheumatoid arthritis, arteriosclerosis, inflammatory bowel disease and Alzheimer's disease (AD).

Exercise increases the rate of oxygen usage, leading several workers to suggest that by-products of increased oxygen consumption, oxygen-derived ROS (Ji et al., 2000), may be responsible for exercise-induced damage to tissue. However, because of these changing redox state, the tissue has developed a number of different mechanisms that adapt rapidly following exercise. These include numerous biochemical changes such as increased activity of antioxidant enzymes, contents of HSPs, and metallothioneins. These adaptations are associated with protection against the potentially damaging effects of exercise.

In this chapter, the beneficial effects of exercise will be interpreted by the hormetic mechanism, which shows that a significant increase in ROS production is rapidly followed by a significant increase in the expression of antioxidant enzymes, metallothioneins, and HSPs, suggesting that a change in redox state of tissue may act as signal for adaptation. We will end with a discussion on beneficial effects of nitric oxide (NO) on both hemodynamic control and metabolic regulation during exercise.

1 Oxidative Stress by Exercise

a) Oxidative stress

Although the implication of ROS in exercise-induced tissue damage appeared in the literature as early as the late 1970s (Jenkins, 1988), the work of Davies et al. (1982) was the first attempt to establish a causal relationship between ROS generation and oxidative cell injury in rodents. Using the electron paramagnetic resonance (EPR) spectroscopy method, they demonstrated that ROS signals are intensified in rat hind limb muscle and liver after an acute bout of treadmill running to exhaustion. Increased ROS production coincided with a series of cellular disorders, such as lipid peroxidation, loss of sarcoplasmic reticulum latency, and mitochondrial uncoupling. Jackson et al. (1985) found a 70% increase in the EPR signals in electrically stimulated contracting muscle. Kumar et al. (1992) showed that an acute bout of exhaustive endurance exercise increased the generation of ROS in the myocardium of female albino rats. Furthermore, lipid peroxidation was increased in the myocardium of these exercised animals.

Reid et al.(1992) adopted 2′,7′-dichlorofluorescin as an intracellular probe to measure reactive oxidant production in contracting diaphragm muscle. They found that ROS, including $\cdot O_2^-$ and H_2O_2, were not only increased during muscle contraction but also might be a contributing factor of low-frequency fatigue in the diaphragm. Despite the limited direct evidence of ROS generation during exercise, there is an abundance of literature providing indirect support that the oxidative process occurs at cellular and molecular levels when oxygen consumption is markedly increased.

When polyunsaturated fatty acids on the biomembrane are attacked by ROS in the presence of molecular oxygen, a chain of peroxidative reactions occurs, eventually leading to the formation of hydrocarbon gases and aldehydes. By-products of lipid peroxidation are the most frequently studied markers of oxidative tissue damage during exercise. Dillard et al. (1978) were the first to show that pentane concentration is increased in the expired gas of human subjects after long-term exercise. Malondialdehyde (MDA) content has been found to increase during exercise in a variety of tissues, and the extent of lipid peroxidation also appears to depend on exercise intensity (Davies et al., 1982; Allessio, 1993).

In addition to lipid peroxidation, ROS are known to cause oxidative modification of proteins and nucleic acid (Stadman, 1990). In rats, a single bout of exhaustive running or endurance training for 12 weeks has been shown to induce a significant increase in protein oxidation of the skeletal muscles (Reznick et al., 1992; Witt et al., 1992). Supplementation of antioxidants attenuated the increase in protein oxidation due to a single bout of exercise, indicating that ROS are involved in the process. Urinary 8-hydroxy deoxyguanosine has recently been used as a marker of steady-state unrepaired DNA levels. DNA damage was found significantly increased after a marathon race (Allessio, 1993). Thus, there seems to be little doubt that excessive exercise can have detrimental effects on cell membrane and structure and may even affect genetic materials.

b) Sources of ROS

The electron transport associated with the mitochondrial respiratory chain is considered the major process leading to ROS production at rest and during exercise. It is widely assumed that during exercise the increased electron flow through the mitochondrial electron transport chain leads to an increased rate of ROS production (Di-Meo and Venditi, 2001). The mitochondrial respiration chain could also be a potential source of ROS in tissues, such as liver, kidney, and nonworking muscles, which during exercise undergo partial ischemia because of reduced blood supply (Di-Meo and Venditi, 2001). Sufficient oxygen is available to interact with the increasingly reduced respiratory chain and enhance the ROS generation. At the cessation of exercise, blood flow to hypoxic tissue resumes leading to their reoxygenation. This mimics the ischemia-reperfusion phenomenon, which is known to cause excessive production of ROS.

Although the mitochondrial respiratory chain is believed to be the major cellular source of ROS production during exercise, a number of alternative pathways have also been proposed. A xanthine oxidase catalyzed reaction occurs in the cytosol and resembles the mechanism of ischemia reperfusion injury (Meydani and Evans, 1993). Under anaerobic conditions due to exhaustive exercise a large amount of ADP would be formed upon ATP depletion in the skeletal muscle. ATP would then be regenerated at the expense of two molecules of ADP by the catalytic action of adenylate kinase, AMP being formed as a byproduct that is metabolized to adenosine and then to hypoxanthine by adenosine deaminase. Hypoxanthine would diffuse out from the muscle into the circulating blood and thereby be provided as a substrate for xanthine oxidase located on the surface of endothelial cells of the lung or in circulation, generating ROS during the enzyme reaction. In support of this interpretation, oxidative stress due to acute exhaustive exercise was shown to be attenuated by the injection of long-lived derivated SOD in spite of a marked increase in xanthine oxidase activity in the plasma (Radak et al., 1995). More recently, Vina et al. (2000) found not only that exercise caused an increase in blood xanthine oxidase activity in rats but also that inhibiting xanthine oxidase with allopurinol prevented exercise-induced oxidation of glutathione (GSH) in both rats and humans.

It is well known that activated blood-borne neutrophils produce $\cdot O_2^-$ and H_2O_2 when they are attracted to the myocytes or the endothelial cells of the vascular beds as a result of muscle cell damage (Meydani and Evans, 1993). Given the time required for neutrophil infiltration, this pathway probably does not explain the acute ROS production and oxidative stress during exercise. However, it may serve as an important secondary source of ROS production and may contribute to the oxidative tissue damage during ultra-endurance sports such as marathon running or the injury after excessive exercise (Zerba et al., 1990).

Peroxidative modification of membrane lipids has been extensively studied and proposed to be a result as well as a major cause of increased oxidant production (Yu, 1994). Biochemical and/or structural defects of membrane lipids may cause further ROS generation *via* the enzymatic pathways involving cyclooxygenase, NADPH oxidase, and xanthine oxidase (Sawada et al., 1992, Chung et al., 1997).

c) Exercise-induced tissue damage through ROS generation

Tissue damage induces a complete cascade of nonspecific events, known as the inflammatory response. The local response involves the production of ROS/RNS and cytokines that are released at the site of inflammation. These ROS/RNS and cytokines facilitate an influx and activation of lymphocytes, neutrophils, monocytes and other cells. These cells participated in the clearance of the antigen and the healing of the tissue. The local inflammatory response is accompanied by a systemic response known as the acute phase response.

A small increase in ROS and cytokines has been found after excessive exercise. However, high levels of ROS and cytokines are associated with exercise causing tissue damage. The close association between the exercise-induced tissue damage and cytokine and ROS responses give rise to an important question: Does damaged tissue initiate the production of ROS and cytokines or do the cytokines induce tissue damage? To answer this question, we hereby put forth a model (Fig.1) for tissue damage and cytokines. In relation to excessive exercise, cells are mechanically damaged leading to necrosis/apoptosis and the initiation of an inflammatory process. Thus, the production of inflammatory cytokines and ROS further stimulate the development of an acute inflammatory response with accumulation in the tissue of neutrophils, followed by macrophages. The cytokines and ROS stimulate infiltrating macrophages to produce prostaglandins, which are central in the sensation of delayed onset pain. Furthermore, the inflammatory cytokines and ROS contribute either directly or indirectly to the prolonged tissue damage.

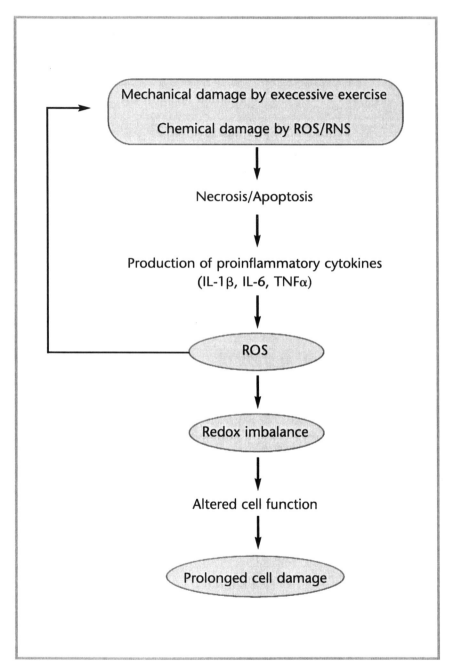

Figure 1. Possible mechanisms of tissue damage by excessive exercise.

2 Changes in the Antioxidative Defense System by Exercise

Mammalian tissues contain enzymatic and nonenzymatic antioxidant defense systems that protect or minimize oxidative tissue damage caused by ROS. Current literature indicates that exercise training can enhance both antioxidant capacity and oxidative capacity in skeletal muscle (Jenkins et al., 1984; Ji et al., 1988; Powers et al., 1992).

An acute bout of exercise is known to increase the activities of antioxidant enzymes, including superoxide dismutase (SOD), catalase, and GSH peroxidase (GPX) in skeletal muscle, heart, and liver (Jenkins, 1988; Ji and Fu, 1992; Ji, 1992). Long term exercise training also appears to increase the activity of several antioxidant enzymes such as SOD, catalase, or GPX in muscle, although these findings are not consistent (Hong and Johnson, 1995; Kim et al., 1996). In humans, exercise training has been reported to increase skeletal muscle SOD activities and the activities of various protective enzymes in blood (Powers et al., 1999; Duthie et al., 1990). The differential effect of training on various antioxidant enzymes may reflect the specific cellular locations where ROS are produced as well as the basal antioxidant capacity in various tissues. Skeletal muscle has one of the lowest antioxidant enzyme levels in the body, but oxygen flux can increase up to several dozen-fold during strenuous exercise (Meydani and Evans, 1993). The resultant large increase in ROS is the likely trigger of antioxidant enzyme synthesis, either directly or indirectly.

3 Exercise and Mitogen-activated Protein Kinase (MAPK)

Exercise training increases muscle mass (Booth and Kiry, 1992; Booth and Thomason, 1991), improves glucose tolerance (Hughes et al., 1993; Rodgers et al., 1988), and increases glucose uptake (Hjeltnes et al., 1998; Rodgers et al., 1988; Wallberg-Henriksson, 1986). These exercise-induced adaptations may be associated with changes in the expression of key proteins involved in metabolism (Chibalin et al., 2000; Hjeltnes et al., 1998; Hughes et al., 1993; Kraniou et al., 2000; Ren et al., 1994). Recent interest has focused on delineating exercise-responsive signaling pathways in skeletal muscle (Aronson, 1997; Goodyear et al., 1996; Widegren et al., 1998). The mitogen-activated protein kinase (MAPK) signaling network regulates gene transcription and protein synthesis (Cano, 1995; Cobb, 1995; Cohen, 1997; Hill and Treisman, 1995), and this may be a possible mechanism by which exercise and muscle contraction lead to increased expression of muscle proteins (Aronson, 1997; Goodyear et al., 1996; Widegren et al., 1998).

The MAPK cascade is a ubiquitously expressed, intracellular network of proteins that forms a major signaling system by which cells transduce extracellular cues into intracellular responses (Seger and Krebs, 1995; Blenis, 1993). The MAPK family includes extracellular-regulated kinase (ERK), c-Jun NH2-terminal kinase (JNK), and p38 MAPK. The classical MAPK enzymes, p42 and p44 ERK, are activated by polypeptide growth factors and tumor-promoting phorbol esters (Cohen, 1997; Hill and Treisman, 1995). JNK and p38 integrate intracellular signals from diverse extracellular stimuli including oxidative stress and heat shock.

Signaling cascades leading to the MAPK pathways are activated in response to muscle contraction. p42/p44 ERK and p38 MAPK are activated in human and rat skeletal muscle by exercise (Aronson, 1997; Goodyear et al., 1996; Widegren et al., 1998). Furthermore, muscle contraction evoked by electrical stimulation leads to the activation of p42/p44 ERK and p38 MAPK (Ryder et al., 2000). Moreover, both p42/p44 ERK and p38 MAPK are phosphorylated in human skeletal muscle in response to exercise (Widegren et al., 1998). However, the pattern of exercise-induced phosphorylation of these two kinases is different (Widegren et al., 1998). Phosphorylation of p42/22 ERK is rapid, restricted to the working muscle, and returnes to basal levels after cessation of exercise. In contrast, p38 MAPK phosphorylation is induced more slowly, and it is not restricted to the exercising muscle, suggesting that systemic factors could play a role in the activation of p38 MAPK. In case of JNK, an acute bout of exercise results in a contraction-dependent stimulation of JNK activity and the induction of its downstream nuclear target c-*Jun* in human skeletal muscle. Moreover, the activation of JNK activity is restricted to the exercising leg (Krook et al., 2000). These results suggest that exercise-induced JNK signaling is an intrinsic response of the contracting muscle rather than a systemic response to exercise.

How does physical exercise cause the activation of the MAPK pathway? One possibility is that MAPK signaling is a function of the exercise-induced increase in blood flow and the corresponding increase in delivery of humoral factors to the muscle, leading to activation of receptor-mediated signaling molecules (Hayashi et al., 1999). Alternatively, the release of neurotransmitters at the neuromuscular junction in the contracting muscles could stimulate cell surface receptors. Because there is evidence for the release of autocrine and paracrine factors from contracting skeletal muscle fibers (Hellsten and Frandsen, 1997; Reid, 1998; Stebbins et al., 1990), these molecules could also play a role in stimulating MAPK signaling. Another possibility is that the contractile activity per se, independent of hormones, neurotransmitters, or autocrine and paracrine factors, increases MAPK signaling in skeletal muscle during physical exercise. Factors that may contribute to the local stimulation of the MAPK pathway by exercise include changes in osmolarity, intracellular calcium levels, or intracellular energy depletion, all of which have been reported to activate MAPK in other cell types (Yoshio et al., 1995; Chao et al., 1994; Bogoyevitch et al., 1995), which might be involved in nuclear factor kappa B (NF-kB) activation, inflammation, or cell growth.

4 Exercise and Redox-sensitive Nuclear Factor Kappa B

Oxidation-reduction (redox)-based regulation of signal transduction and gene expression is emerging as a fundamental regulatory mechanism in cell biology (Sen and Packer, 1996; Sen, 1998). In mammalian cells, the redox sensitive transcription factor NF-κB has been well defined (Sen and Packer, 1996; Sen, 1998). In most cell types, NF-κB mediates an immediate early response by activating the transcription of numerous genes encoding pro-inflammatory proteins, such as cell adhesion molecules, cytokines, and chemokines.

GSH plays a central role in the maintenance of tissue antioxidant defense and in the regulation of redox-sensitive signal transduction. Intracellular thiol redox status appears to be a critical determinant of NF-κB activation. At low levels of cytosolic GSSG, T-cells fail to activate NF-κB in response to appropriate stimuli, whereas high GSSG concentration inhibits the binding of activated NF-κB to its cognate DNA site. Thus, it appears that an intermediate optimal level of intracellular GSSG is required for effective NF-κB activation. Droge et al. (1994) found that GSH deficiency of T-cell is associated with a suppression of NF-κB function.

In muscle cells, the level and redox status of GSH regulates activity of the redox sensitive transcription factor NF-κB. Physical exercise may cause oxidation of GSH in tissues such as the skeletal muscle and liver (Sen and Hanninen, 1994). Lew et al (1985) reported that exhaustive exercise decreases both liver and muscle GSH consistently . Elevated skeletal muscle GSSG/GSH ratios have been observed in physiological oxidative stress situations such as those triggered by strenuous exercise (Sen, 1995) or immobilization (Kondo and Itokawa, 1994).

Tumor necrosis factor α (TNFα) is a cytokine product of monocytes and macrophages (Akira et al., 1990). It has been shown that exhaustive exercise by athletes results in increased TNFα levels in the serum (Weinstock et al., 1997), suggesting that TNFα may be implicated in exhaustive exercise-induced muscle damage. Sen et al. (1997) investigated the role of endogenous GSH status in TNFα -induced NF-κB activation in skeletal muscle-derived cells. In GSH deficient cells, TNFα-induced NF-κB activation was potentiated, suggesting that such activation is sensitive to cellular GSH (Sen et al., 1997). Enhancement of cell GSH inhibited TNFα -induced NF-κB activation (Sen et al., 1997). Conditions such as lowered cellular GSH level or elevated cellular GSSG levels that were observed to potentiate TNFα-induced NF-κB activation may be expected to contribute to muscle pathologies including the development of cachexic processes in TNFα-exposed skeletal muscle tissue. NF-κB activation might be regulated by the GSSG/GSH ratio which is changed during exercise.

5 Changes in NF-κB and Cytokines in Inflammatory Diseases

An intricate relationship exists among NF-κB, inflammation, and oxidative stress such that NF-κB regulation is exquisitely sensitive to ROS and the redox status (Chung et al., 2000). The NF-κB family has been identified in various organisms ranging from flies to mammals, and is known to play a central role in various responses that lead to a host of defenses through rapid gene expression induction. In particular, NF-κB also controls the expression of various inflammatory cytokines (Fox et al., 1996), cell adhesion molecules (Yan et al., 1999), immunoreceptors (Kwon, 2000), and acute-phase proteins.

NF-κB regulates immune reactions, inflammation, cell proliferation, carcinogenesis, and apoptosis through gene expression. Redox-sensitive NF-κB regulates the transcription of numerous genes involved in cellular inflammatory responses. NF-κB has been shown to modulate the expression of gene coding for TNFα, IL-1β, IL-6, MHC class I antigens, and serum amyloid A precursor (Tanaka et al., 1997). During inflammatory reactions, many genes are turned on as needed by the organism. Under challenged conditions from bacteria, viruses, or physical and chemical stressors, proinflammatory genes activate and their encoded proteins are expressed. The newly synthesized proteins by NF-κB serve to defend the organism and to put it into a stage of alert. Many are signaling proteins, such as cytokines, growth factors, or chemokines, which stimulate the immune system. Some are mediators that enable cells to better respond to growth-stimulation or apoptopic signals.

Although the involvement of the inflammatory process in several major diseases is long known, its implication in the aging process has been less appreciated until a recent proposal by McGeer et al. in their "Inflammatory Hypothesis of Dementia" (McGeer et al., 1999). Neurological disorders such as Parkinson's disease and Alzheimer's disease (AD) are now well established to be characterized by ROS formation. In addition to direct attacks on neurons, ROS may function as signaling molecules for the modulation of NF-κB. For instance, Kaltschmidt et al. (1997) reported that amyloid β-peptides , a hallmark of AD, induces significant NF-κB activity, which requires ROS as messengers. NF-κB activation leads to transcriptional activation of many genes that may contribute to neurodegenerative and inflammatory conditions as with AD (Goto et al., 1999).

Ample evidence shows that the inflammatory process underlies major vascular diseases (Thomas et al., 1999). For example, age-related inflammatory processes are well exemplified in the age-related alterations of vascular endothelial and smooth muscle cells, which lead to pathogenic expressions as seen in atherosclerosis (Collins, 1993), and the vascular degeneration caused by diabetes (Oberley, 1998).

Vascular endothelial cells (EC) form an interface between tissues and plasma. This unique localization exposes EC to external stresses. As a consequence of stress or injury, EC initiate appropriate physiological responses to maintain normal vascular tone and blood flow, which is usually accompanied by increases in vascular permeability induction of a prothrombogenic surface and the stimulation of leukocyte extravasation. Given their central role in the initiation and coordination of inflammatory responses, EC play a primary role in the pathogenesis of many systemic inflammation processes (Whicher et al., 1999).

Cytokines, such as TNFα, IL-1β, and INF-α, produce vascular leaks through cytoskeletal reorganization within EC, that result in delayed but persistent increases in vascular permeability. In animal studies, a TNFα or INFβ injection resulted in local swelling of microvascular EC in the vessel wall, which indicates increased vascular permeability (Papadaki et al., 1999). Incubation with lipopolysaccharide (LPS), a potent immune stimulate, resulted in direct morphologic changes in bovine EC, including dilation of intracellular junctions, cell contraction, and ruffling of the surface membrane (Famaey, 1982). The activities of cytokines and other proinflammatory agents likely cause microvascular alteration, leading to enhanced permeability and to a full, clinical inflammatory response.

6 Cytokine and Exercise

The first study to suggest that exercise induces a cytokine response reported that plasma obtained from human subjects after exercise, and injected intraperitoneally into rats, elevated rectal temperature (Cannon et al., 1983). In 1986, two studies were published that indicated that the level of IL-1β increased in response to exercise (Cannon et al.,1986). An increase in IL-6 concentration was reported immediately after a marathon run, but there was no detectable IL-1β (Evans et al., 1986). IL-6 was also shown to be elevated in response to exercise (Castell et al, 1997). Several studies have failed to detect TNF-α after exercise (River et al., 1994), whereas others reported increased plasma TNF-α concentrations (Espersen et al., 1990). There are several possible explanations for the variable results on pro-inflammatory and inflammation-responsive cytokines in relation to exercise (Pedersen, 1998). These include the type of physical activity as well as the intensity and duration of the exercise. Increased cytokine levels have been described mostly after execessive exercise. The magnitude of the increase is probably related to the duration of the exercise, although this remains to be shown in studies comparing cytokine levels in groups of subjects performing exercise at same intensity but at varying durations. Initially, IL-6 was thought to be a pro-inflammatory cytokine but recent results have suggested that IL-6 has an inflammation-controlling function and is important for the return to homeostasis after an inflammatory challenge (Tilg et al., 1997; Xing et al., 1998). Plasma IL-6 concentration has been found to be elevated in a variety of conditions where system homeostasis is threatened or compromised, such as in sepsis or with multiple trauma (Hack et al., 1997; Giannoudis et al., 1998). Interestingly, recent findings have shown strenuous exercise is also a powerful inducer of elevated concentrations of IL-6 in plasma (Drenth et al., 1995; Castell et al., 1997; Nehlsen-Cannarella et al., 1997; Osrowski et al., 1998a, b, 1999). In a previous study, involving trained athletes running on a treadmill for 2.5h, a strong positive correlation was found between the peak plasma IL-6 concentration reached at the end of running and the plasma lactate concentration at the same time-point (Osrowski et al., 1998b). This led us to the idea that the concentration of IL-6 could be related to either the running intensity or the duration of exercise (Jacobs, 1986). Furthermore, it is noted that marathon running resulted in a 100-fold increase in plasma IL-6 concentration (Osrowski et al. 1999), whereas a less strenuous (shorter duration and slightly lower intensity) treadmill run resulted in only a 25-fold increase (Osrowski et al., 1998b). On the other hand, the expression of the antioxidant and anti-apoptotic factors metallothionein I+II (MT-I+II) was increased prominently by the freeze lesion, but this response was significantly reduced in the IL-6-deficient (Knockout, IL-6 KO) mice. By contrast, the expression of the antioxidants Cu/Zn-superoxide dismutase (Cu/Zn-SOD), Mn-SOD, and catalase remained unaffected by the IL-6 deficiency (Milena et al., 2000). The changes in tissue damage and in the regeneration observed in IL-6KO mice are likely caused by the IL-6-dependent decrease in MT-I+II expression, indicating IL-6 and MT-I+II as neuroprotective factors during tissue injury.

7 Heat Shock Proteins, Metallothioneins and Exercise

a) Induction of heat shock proteins by exercise

Heat shock proteins (HSP) are cell-protective and antioxidant systems that may be induced by ROS, cytokines, and hyperthermia. Exercise-induced alterations indicate that immunocompetent cells become activated. In addition to heat stress, other exercise-associated stress agents (oxidants, cytokines) may participate in the stimulation of HSP expression in leukocytes. The expression pattern of HSP due to training status may be attributed to adaptive mechanisms. Regular endurance training seems to affect protective mechanisms beneficially in immunocompetent cells. The enhanced heat shock response in the athletes at rest may represent an activation of the protective resources in immune cells from denaturing heat. This may be interpreted as a training-induced adaptive mechanism or as an acquired thermotolerance (Fehrenbach et al., 1999). Exercise-induced oxidant, cytokine, and heat stress may be involved in the stress response. These results are potentially valid to monitor beneficial or unfavorable effects of intensive endurance exercise or extensive training and to estimate the relevance of individual stress gene responses in circulating leukocytes.

Many generated stress conditions can result, at the molecular level, in the rapid production of HSPs, stress proteins with the chaperone function of maintaining and repairing protein conformation. Despite the name, these proteins are implicated not only in the protection of cells from heat stress, but also against different types of proteotoxic insults such as oxidative stress, exposure to amino acid analogs, heavy metals, and others (Locke et al., 1990). Thus HSP expression could represent an important protective mechanism against exercise-induced damage to muscle. It was shown that sedentary rats submitted to a bout of intense exercise have increased muscular expression of HSP72 after a period of 2 h (Niess et al., 1999), indicating that HSP72 is rapidly synthesized in response to exercise stress. Moreover, ischemia-reperfusion studies of the cardiac muscle provide evidence for the direct role of HSP72 in the prevention of oxidative-stress damage in this tissue (Mosser et al., 1993). It is suggested that HSP72 may represent an important protective mechanism against oxidative damage to proteins caused by ROS. The involvement of HSP72 (and other HSPs) in the antioxidant defense system is still unclear, and this involvement certainly needs to be better analyzed. It is possible that the regulation of HSP72 expression is important in muscle resistance to exercise stress.

b) Induction of metallothioneins by exercise

Metallothioneins occur throughout the animal kingdom and they are induced in vivo by metals, hormones, cytotoxic agents, and some kind of stress. It is well known that various stresses such as starvation and immobilization can induce metallothionein synthesis in animal tissues (Shinogi et al., 1999). It is reported that the levels of metallothionein were decreased by 13-34% in lung, liver, heart and skeletal muscle of rats trained by swimming for 10 weeks and were increased by 21%-75% in skeletal muscle, heart, brain, lung, and liver of rats after exhaustive swimming, compared with normal control rats. It is suggested that the different changes of metallothionein levels under physical training and acute exhaustive exercise may be of importance in the protection against ROS.

8 Management of Inflammatory Diseases by Dietary Restriction and Exercise

DR (DR, reduced calorie intake) can increase the neuronal resistance to dysfunction and death in experimental models of Alzheimer's disease, Parkinson's disease, Huntington's disease and stroke. The mechanism underlying the beneficial effects of DR involves the stimulation of the expression of stress proteins and neurotrophic factors. The neurotrophic factors induced by DR may protect neurons by inducing the production of proteins that suppress oxyradical production, stabilize cellular calcium homeostasis and inhibit apoptotic biochemical cascades (Mattson 2000). Interestingly, DR also increases the number of newly generated neural cells in the adult brain suggesting that this dietary manipulation can increase the brain's capacity for plasticity and self-repair. It is suggested that physical and intellectual activity can similarly increase neurotrophic factor production and neurogenesis (Mattson, 2000). Collectively, the available data suggest that DR, as well as physical and mental activity, may reduce both the incidence and severity of neurodegenerative disorders in humans. A better understanding of the cellular and molecular mechanisms underlying these effects of diet and behavior on the brain is also leading to novel therapeutic agents that mimic the beneficial effects of DR and exercise. DR is shown to significantly increase spontaneous locomotive activity, which suggests that the beneficial effects of DR are associated with exercise effect (Yu et al., 1985). Futhermore, Chung et al. (2001) reported that DR showed an anti-inflammatory action during the aging process.

Significant improvements in muscle strength, oxygen and well-being were found in patients with inflammatory myopathy, polymyositis, and dermatomyositis as a result of physical training (Wiesinger et al., 1998). A physically active lifestyle has been shown to be effective in lowering all-cause mortality in the able-bodied population. On the other hand, exercise to the limit of claudication leads to local and systemic inflammatory response. Concerns that exercise training leads to the progression of atherosclerosis from inflammation are misplaced. Such training causes attenuation of inflammation and improves blood rheological properties. Furthermore, the effect of training may be analogous to the biological response associated with myocardial ischaemic preconditioning (Tan, et al., 2000). Exercise training leads to a reduction in the oxygen cost of exercise, a higher peak oxygen utilization and a reduction in heart rate, representing an improvement in the cardiorespiratory status of the patient (Tan, et al., 2000). An exercise program frequently improves both the physical and quality aspects of life, and the success of an exercise program is multifactorial. An increase in the blood flow to the lower extremity is uncommon. The changes that do seem to occur such as a redistribution of blood flow, changes in oxidative capacity of the skeletal muscles, and greater utilization of oxygen are those that lead to a rectification of the associated metabolic dysfunction of the skeletal muscle. Following exercise training, blood rheology improves and exercise-induced inflammation is ameliorated; cardiorespiratory status also benefits and the oxygen cost of exercise decrease (Tan, et al., 2000). There beneficial effects of exercise appears to be due to physiological nitric oxide (NO) released by exercise training, which might lead to improvement in the above referenced cardiovascular inflammatory diseases.

9 Exercises and NO

a) Induction of endothelial NOS by exercise

Nitric oxide (NO) mediates many physiologic processes including immune, inflammatory, nervous, cardiovascular, and pulmonary systems. NO is generated by NO synthase (NOS) through a series of complex redox reaction steps (Nathan and Xie, 1994a) utilizing molecular oxygen and the guanidine nitrogen of arginine as the substrates, NADPH (Marietta, 1993; Tsao et al., 1990) as an electron donor, and flavine adenine dinucleotide, flavine mononucleotide, heme, tetrahydrobiopterin, and Ca^{2+}/calmodulin as cofactors (Rufahl et al., 1992; Stuehr et al., 1991; Marietta, 1994).

NOS is classified into three isotypes (McDonald and Murad, 1996; Fostermann and Kleinert, 1995; Pollock, 1995). Type I NOS, also called neuronal NOS or brain constitutive NOS (bNOS) (Bredit et al., 1991), is an isozyme found in high concentration in some neuronal cells (Nathan and Xia, 1994b; Bredit and Snyder, 1992; Nathan, 1992; Bredit et al., 1990). The isozyme is activated by calmodulin when intracellular Ca^{2+} is elevated. Type II NOS is referred to as macrophage NOS or inducible NOS (Nathan and Xia, 1994b; Nathan, 1992). This enzyme is not present in un-stimulated, resting cells, but can be induced in a number of cell types by exposure to bacteria, and lipopolysaccharides in conjunction with cytokines (Nathan and Xia, 1994b). This isozyme is normally independent of Ca^{2+} activation. Type II NOS induction is probably a part of the mechanism for mounting a cytotoxic response (Fostermann and Kleinert, 1995). Type III NOS, also known as endothelial constitutive NOS (eNOS) (Marsden et al., 1993; Miyahara et al., 1994; Sessa et al., 1992; Janssens et al., 1992), is the isoform commonly associated with production of endothelium-derived relaxing factor (EDRF) (Nathan, 1992). Like type I NOS, this isozyme is activated by intracellular Ca^{2+} concentration and calmodulin binding to the enzyme (Bredit and Snyder, 1990). eNOS is most abundant in aorta, heart, lung, kidney, adrenal gland, spinal cord, and urogenital tissues.

Physical conditioning is known to increase expiratory NO output during exercise (Maroun et al., 1995). Furthermore, exercise is likely to affect the vasomotor function of the skeletal muscle and vessels that have an important role in the regulation of peripheral resistance (Dong et al., 1994). During exercise, several factors may affect the regulation of arteriolar resistance. One of the main characteristics of exercise is that it reduces resistance so that blood flow greatly increases to skeletal muscles to meet the increase in metabolic demand (Armstrong et al., 1984; Kjellmer, 1964; Laughlin and Armstrong, 1982; Musch and Terrell, 1992). Regular exercise can induce both structural and functional changes in the peripheral vascular system, in the regulation of peripheral resistance and in skeletal muscle metabolism. The development of these beneficial changes was shown to be dependent on both the intensity and duration of exercise. Although the NO's involvement in exercise-induced vasodilation (Koller et al., 1998; Kane et al., 1994) is firmly established, for instance, the study of Zhao et al. (1997) showed that short-term exercise training enhances the release of NO from the endothelial cells, and Woodman et al. (1997) showed an upregulation of eNOS gene expression by exercise training in porcine coronary resistance arteries.

NO is known to have a potent influence on renal function though both renal hemodynamic and tubular effects. It assures adequate oxygenation of the renal medulla (Zou et al., 1998) and regulates glomerular capillary pressure. NO produced by endothelial cells can inhibit sodium transport by cortical collecting duct cells. Chronic NOS inhibition has been reported to reduce blood flow in the renal medullary circulation (Mattson et al., 1997), which could secondarily influence sodium and water excretion by altering physical factors.

In a dog study, Sessa et al. (1994) showed that chronic exercise (i.e. running on a treadmill 9.5 Km/h for 1 hr, twice daily for 10 days) enhanced NO production and endothelial NOS expression in the aorta. Exercise also stimulates c-Jun NH2 Kinase activity and c-Jun transcriptional activity in human skeletal muscle. To assess the effect of exercise on gene expression, a recent rat study determined mRNA levels and protein of eNOS by RT-PCR and Western blotting. The mRNA levels in exercised rats were markedly increased compared to the control group, and the extent of increase was dependent on the duration of exercise (Huh et al., 1999). Protein levels of eNOS which shows a denatured molecular mass of 135 kDa (Fostermann and Kleinert, 1995) were in parallel to mRNA level. These results were consistent with previous studies which exercise increased vascular NO production and eNOS gene expression (Uematsu et al., 1995; Sessa et al., 1994).

Endothelial release of NO is stimulated by numerous hormones (e.g., acetylcholine and bradykinin) and by mechanical stimuli (shear stress) (Furchgott and Vanhoutte, 1989; Rubanyi et al., 1986). Although many stimuli are known to regulate NOS activity acutely, few factors are known to regulate endothelial NOS gene expression. Shear stress is known to increase endothelial NOS mRNA and protein (Ninchida et al., 1992), whereas TNF-α decreases NOS mRNA post-transcriptionally (Yoshizumi et al., 1993).

Furthermore, Uematsu et al. (1995) reported that exposure of endothelial cells to chronic shear stress enhances expression of mRNA and protein of NO synthase as well as produces NO in bovine aortic endothelial cells. Sun et al. (1998) suggested that during the periods of exercise activity the intermittent increase in blood flow/shear stress in arterioles of skeletal muscle may be the underlying mechanism responsible for flow-induced dilation of arterioles.

In conclusion, it is suggested that eNOS gene expression is induced by regular and adapted exercise, and that it may help to explain the beneficial effects of physical exercise on the regulation of blood circulation.

b) Exercise as a stimulus for NO

NO is implicated in such diverse processes as vasodilation, inhibition of platelet aggregation, immune function, cell growth, neurotransmission, metabolic regulation and excitation– contraction coupling. Neuronal (n) and endothelial (e) NOS isoforms that produce NO as a signaling mechanism. In humans, in addition to its expression in endothelial cells, eNOS is found in smooth and cardiac muscle, male and female reproductive tracts and brain, while nNOS is expressed in brain, spinal cord, sympathetic ganglia, peripheral nerves, pancreas, epithelial cells of the stomach, lung and uterus and, importantly, skeletal muscle (Chao et al., 1996). From a functional perspective, emphasis will be placed on the role of NO in haemodynamic and metabolic control during exercise, the adaptations that occur with training, and how these may contribute to the preventative and therapeutic effects associated with physical activity and fitness.

Accumulating animal and human data suggest that NO is important for both coronary and peripheral haemodynamic control and metabolic regulation during the performance of exercise. While still controversial, NO of endothelial origin is thought to potentiate exercise-induced hyperemia, both in the peripheral and coronary circulations. The mechanism of release may include both acetylcholine, derived from the neuromuscular junction and vascular shear stress. Exercise training in healthy individuals promotes adaptations in the various NO systems, which can increase NO bioavailability through a variety of mechanisms, including increased NOS enzyme expression and activity. Such adaptations likely contribute to increased exercise capacity and protection from cardiovascular events. Exercise training in individuals with elevated cardiovascular risk or established disease can increase NO bioavailability, which may represent an important mechanism by which exercise training provides benefit as a secondary prevention.

There is increasing evidence that NO is an important haemodynamic and metabolic regulator during the performance of physical activity. Furthermore, there are adaptations in body system as a result of exercise training that likely contribute to increased functional capacity and the cardioprotective effects associated with higher fitness levels. Exercise has particular efficacy in restoring dysfunction of the vascular endothelial NO system, which is becoming established as a precursor to the atherosclerotic process (Cannon et al., 1998). Animal data suggest that this benefit may extend to skeletal muscle NO, which appears, among other functions, to mediate glucose uptake during exercise (Balon et al., 1994).

The intermittent increase in blood flow/shear stress in arterioles of skeletal muscle during the periods of exercise activity may be the underlying mechanism responsible for the adaptation. In large coronary vessels Sessa et al. (1994) showed that these changes are paralleled by an enhanced eNOS gene expression. A study further demonstrated that chronic presence of high blood flow increases aortic eNOS expression (Nadaud et al., 1996). Thus, it is quite likely that the mechanism responsible for the sensing of and responses to increases in blood flow (shear stress) in arterioles may undergo an adaptation, especially in those arterioles that are exposed to great increases in blood flow during exercise.

NO-independent vasodilation causes increased shear stress within the blood vessel which, in turn, stimulates eNOS activation, NO release and the prolongation of vasodilation (Gattullo et al., 1999). Reactive hyperemia, myogenic vasodilation and vasodilator effects of acetylcholine and bradykinin are all mediated by NO. Exercise increases NO synthesis *via* increases in shear stress and pulse pressure, and so it is likely that NO is an important blood flow regulatory mechanism during exercise (Gattullo et al., 1999). This phenomenon may account for the beneficial effects of exercise seen in atherosclerotic individuals. Whilst NO plays a protective role in preventing atherosclerosis via superoxide anion scavenging, risk factors such as hypercholesterolemia reduces NO release, leading to the way for endothelial dysfunction and atherosclerotic lesions (Gattullo et al., 1999). Exercise might reverse this process by stimulating NO synthesis and release.

Shear stress acts as a stimulus for the endothelium to increase the transport capacity for L-arginine (the precursor molecule for NO), to enhance NO synthase activity and expression, and to increase the production of extracellular SOD, which prevents the premature breakdown of NO (Kein et al., 1998). Exercise also affects the microcirculation, where it sensitizes resistance arteries for the vasodilatory effects of adenosine. These findings provide a pathophysiological framework to explain the improvement of myocardial perfusion in the absence of changes in baseline coronary artery diameter (Gattullo et al., 1999). Because endothelial dysfunction has been identified as a predictor of coronary events, exercise may contribute to the long-term reduction of cardiovascular morbidity and mortality.

Levels of vasoactive peptides such as adrenomedullin (AM), endothelin-1 (ET-1), C-type natriuretic peptide (CNP), and NO are affected by fluid shear stress. AM, a potent vasodilator and suppressor of smooth muscle cell proliferation, contains the shear stress responsive element (SSRE), "GAGACC" in its promoter region (Shinoki et al., 1998). These findings suggest that the rapid production of NO by human bone cells in response to fluid flow results from the activation of eNOS. Blood fluid flow also leads to an increase in eNOS mRNA, which is likely related to the shear stress responsive element in the promoter of eNOS (Fig. 2).

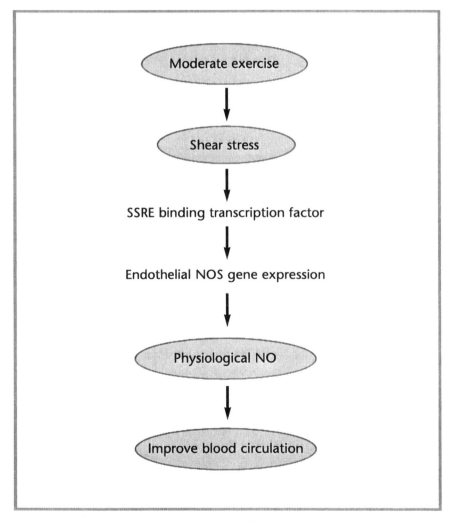

Figure 2. Possible mechanisms of beneficial effects by moderate exercise.

10 Conclusion: Hormetic Mechanism of Exercise

The concept of hormesis originally noted that many types of chemicals stimulated the growth of lower organisms at low doses but inhibited their growth at high doses (Sagan, 1989). Thus, their dose-effect curve would be J-shaped rather than linear. Recently the term hormesis was coined to refer to beneficial effects of low dose of potentially harmful substances. Recent data suggest that the hormesis may operate among higher animals as well (Calabrese et al., 1998). In fact, many researchers suggest that the hormesis concept is a general phenomenon that operates over a wide range of organisms and exposures (Stebbing, 1982).

In addition, Arking et al. (2001) proposed that exposure to a wide variety of stressors will hormetically raise the transient basal level of expression of antioxidant defense system genes and, probably to a lesser extent, HSP genes in the long lived subset of the exposed population.

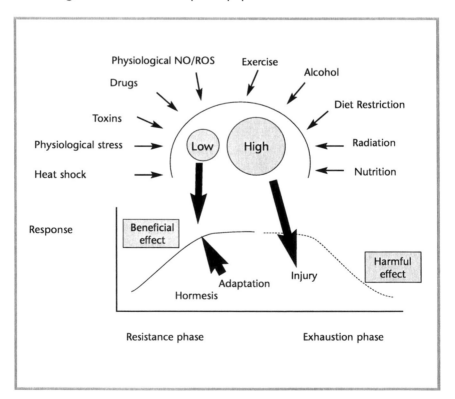

Figure 3. Hormetic Mechanism by Multiple Stimuli.

On the other hand, exercise is also becoming recognized as a stimuli of hormesis. Moderate exercise have well-established beneficial effects, including improved cardiopulmonary function, lower psychosocial stress, and enhancement of the immune system. However, excessive exercise is associated with cardiovascular accidents, joint injuries and immune suppression. (Himeno et al., 2001). It is well-known that average and maximum life spans were extended by CR which is the most effective life-prolonging intervention an evolutionary adapted measure and has resistive action against stress. (Yu and Chung 2001). Interestingly, the CR animals were more active than *adlibitum* group (Yu et al., 1985). The CR effect might be combined with an exercise effect. The evidence strongly suggests that an organisms adaptive response to exercise was acquired through evolution by its ability to activate the proper genes essential for a high metabolically efficient state for survival of species and ROS. The maintenance of homeostasis in organisms may be due to diverse adaptations to environmental stress based on a hormesis-type mechanism, which allows low or moderate levels of stimulus such as exercise to stimulate the production of physiological levels of NO and ROS (Fig. 3).

Acknowledgement
This work was supported by a grant from the Korean Research Foundation (FS 0004).

REFERENCES

Akira, S., Hirano, T., Taga, T., Kishimoto, T. (1990). Biology of multifunctional cytokines: IL-6 and related molecules (IL-1 and TNF). *The Faseb Journal* 4:2860-2867.

Allessio, H.M. (1993). Exercise-induced oxidative stress. *Medicine Science in Sports and Exercise* 25:218-224.

Arking, R. (2001). Antioxidant genes, hormesis, and demographic longevity. *Journal of Antiaging Medicine* (In press).

Armstrong, R.B., Laughlin, H.M. (1984). Exercise blood flow patterns within and among rat muscles after training. *American Journal of Physiology* 246:H59-H68.

Aronson, D., Dufresne, S.D., Goodyear, L.J. (1997). Contratile activity stimulates the c-Jun NH2 –terminal kinase pathway in rat skeletal muscle. *Journal of Biological Chemistry* 272:25636-25640.

Aronson, D., Violan, M.A., Dufresne, S.D., Zangen, D., Fielding, R.A., Goodyear, L.J. (1997). Exercise stimulates the mitogenic-activated protein kinase pathway in human skeletal muscle. *Journal of Clinical Investigation* 99:1251-1257.

Balon T, Nadler J. (1994). Nitric oxide release is present from incubated skeletal muscle preparations. *Journal of Applied Physiology* 77:2519–21.

Blenis, J. (1993). Signal transduction via the MAP kinase: proceed at our own RSK. *Proceeding of National Academy Science USA* 90:5889-5892.

Bogoyevitch, M.A., Ketterman, A.J., Sugden, P.H. (1995). Cellular stresses differentially activate c-Jun N-terminal protein kinases and extracellular signal-regulated protein kinases in cultures ventricular myocytes. *Journal of Biological Chemistry* 270:29710-29717.

Booth, F.W, Kiry, C.R. (1992). Changes in skeletal muscle gene expression consequent to altered weight bearing. American Journal of Physiology. *Regulatory Integrative Comparative Physiology* 262:R239-R332.

Booth, F.W., Thomason, D.B. (1991). Molecular and cellular adaptation of muscle in response to exercise: perspectives of various models. *Physiology Review* 71:541-585.

Bredit, D.S., Hwang, P.M., Glatt, C.E., Lowenstein, C., Reed, R.R., Snyder, S.H. (1991). Cloned and expressed nitric oxide synthase structurally resembles cytochrome P-450 reductase. *Nature* 351:714-718.

Bredt, D.S., Hwang, P.M., Synder, S.H. (1990). Localization of nitric oxide synthase indicating a neuronal role for nitric oxide. *Nature* 347:768-769.

Bredt, D.S., P.M., Synder, S.H. (1992). Nitric oxide a novel neuronal messenger. *Neuron* 8:3-11.

Calabrese, E.J, Baldwin, I.A. (1988). Hormesis as a biological hypothesis. *Environmental Health Perspect* 106:357-362.

Cannon, J.G., Kluger, M.J. (1983). Endogenous pyrogen activity in human plasma after exercise. *Science* 220:617-619.

Cannon, J.G., Evans, W.J, Hughes, V.A., Meredlth, C.N., Dinarello, C.A. (1986). Physiological mechanisms contributing to increased interleukin-1 secretion. *Journal of Applied Physiology* 61:1869-1874.

Cannon, J.G., Orencole, S.F., Fielding, R.A., Meydani, M., Meydani, S.N., Fiatarone M.A., Blumberg, J.B., Evans, W.J. (1990). Acute phase response in exercise: interaction of age and vitamin E on neutrophils and muscle enzyme release. American Journal of of Physiology. *Regulatory Integrative Comparative Physiology* 259:R1214-R1219.

Cannon, R. (1998). Role of nitric oxide in cardiovascular disease: Focus on the endothelium. *Clinical Chemistry* 44:1809–19.

Cano, E., Mahadevan, L.C. (1995). Parallel signal processing among mammalian MAPs. *Trends in Biochemical Science* 20:117-122.

Castell, L.M., Poortmans J.R., Leclercoq, R., Brasseur, M., Duchaterau, J., Newsholme E.A. (1997). Some aspects of the acute phase response after a marathon race, and the effects of glutamine supplementation. *European Journal of Applied Physiology* 75:47-53.

Castell, L.M., Poortmans, J.R., Leclercq, R., Brasseur, M., Duchateru, J., Newsholme E.A. (1997). Some aspects of the acute phase response after a marathon race, and the effects of glutamine supplementation. *European Journal of Applied Phsiology* 75:47-53.

Chao, D., Hwang, P., Huang, F, Bredt, D. (1996). Localization of neuronal nitric oxide synthase. *Methods Enzymology* 268:488–96.

Chao, T.S., Foster, D.A., Rapp, U.R., Rosner, M.R. (1994). Differential Raf requirement for activation of mitogen-activated protein kinase by growth factors, phorbol esters, and calcium. *Journal of Biological Chemistry* 269:7337-7341.

Chibalin, A.V., Yu, M., Ryder, J.W., Song, X.M., Galuska, D., Krook, A., Wallberg-Henriksson, H., Zierath, J.R. (2000). Exercise-induced changes in expression and activity of proteins involved in insulin-signal-transduction in skeletal muscle: differential effects on IRS-1 and IRS-2. *Proceeding of National Academy Science USA* 97:38-43.

Chung, H.Y., Baek, B.S., Song, S.H., Kim, M.S., Huh J.I. (1997). Xanthine dehydrogenase/Xanthine oxidase and oxidative stress. *Age* 20:127-40.

Chung, H.Y., Kim, H.J., Jung, K.J., Yoon, J.S., Yoo, M.A., Kim, K.W., Yu, B.P. (2000). The inflammatory process in aging. *Review Clinical Gerontology* 10:207-222.

Cobb, M.H., Goldsmith, E.J. (1995). How MAP kinases are regulated. *Journal of Biological Chemistry* 270:14843-14846.

Cohen P. (1997). The search for physiological substrates of MAP and SAP kinases in mamallian cells. *Trends in Cell Biology* 7:353-361.

Collins, T. (1993). Endotherial nuclear factor-kappa B and the initiation of the atherosclerotic lesion. *Laboratory Investigation* 68:499-508.

Cuenda A., Rouse J., Doza Y., Meier R., Cohen P., Gallagher T., Young P., Lee J. (1995). Homologue which is stimulated by cellular stresses and interlukin-1. *FEBS Letter* 364:229-323.

Davies, K.J.A., Quintanilha, T.A., Brooks, G.A., Packer, L. (1982). Free radical and tissue damage produced by exercise. *Biochemical and Biophysical Research Communications* 107:1198-1205.

Dillard, C.J., Litov, R.E., Savin, W.M., Dumclin, E.E., Tapple, A.L. (1978). Effect of exercise, vitamin E, and ozone on pulmonary function and lipid peroxidation. *Journal of Applied Physiology* 45:927-932.

Di-Meo, S., Venditi, P. (2001). Mitochondria in exercise-induced oxidative stress. *Biological Signals and Receptors* 10:125-140.

Dong, S., Huang, A., Koller, A., Kaley, G. (1994). Short-term daily exercise activity enhances endothelial NO synthesis in skeletal muscle arterioles of rats. *Journal of Applied Physiology* 75:2241-2247.

Drenth, J.P., Uum, S.H., van, Deuren, M., van, Pesman, G.J., Der Ven Jongekrijg, J van, Der Meer JWM van. Endurance run increases circulating IL-6 and IL-1ra but downregulates ex vivo TNF-α and IL-I beta production. *Journal of Applied Physiology* 79:1497-1503.

Droge, W., Schulze-Osthoff, K., Mihm, S., Galter, D., Schenk, H., Eck, H.P., Roth, S., Gmunder, H. (1994). Functions of glutathione and glutathione disulfide in immunology and immunopathology. *The FASEB Journal* 8:1131-1138.

Duthie, G.G., Robertson, J.D., Maughan, R.J., Morrice, P.C. (1990). Blood antioxidant status and erythrocyte lipid peroxidation following distance running. *Archives of Biochemistry and Biophysics* 282:78-83.

Espersen, G.T., Elbaek, A., Ernst, E., Toft, E., Kaalund, S., Jersild C., Grunnet, N. (1990). Effect of physical exercise on cytokines and lymphocyte subpopulations in human peripheral blood. *Acta Pathologica, Microbiologica, et Immunologica Scandinavica* 98:395-400.

Evans, W.J., Meredith, C.N., Cannon, J.G., Dinarello, C.A., Fronterra, W.R., Hughes, V.A, Jonses, B.H., Knuttgen, H.G. (1986). Metabolic changes following eccentric exercise in trained and untrained men. *Journal of Applied Physiology* 61:1864-1868.

Famaey, J.P. (1982). Free radicals and activated oxygen. *European Journal of Rhumatology and Inflammation* 5:350-59.

Fehrenbach, E, and Niess, A.M. (1999). Role of heat shock proteins in the exercise response. *Exercise Immunology Review* 5:57-77.

Flanagan, S.W., Ryan, A.J., Gisolfi, C.V., Moseley, P.L. (1995). Tissue-specific HSP70 response in animals undergoing heat stress. *American Journal of Physiology. Regulatory Integrative Comparative Physiology* 268:R28-R32.

Forstermann, U., Tracey, W.R., Nakane, M. (1995). Nitric oxide synthase isozymes anti-bodies. *The Histochemical Journal* 27:738-741.

Fox, E.S., Cantrell, C.H., Leingang, K.A. (1996). Inhibition of the Kupffer cell inflammatory response by acute ethanol: NF-kappa B activation and subsequent cytokine production. *Biochemical and Biophysical Research Communications* 225:134-40.

Gattullo, D., Pagliaro, P., Marsh, N.A., Losano, G. (1999). New insights into nitric oxide and coronary circulation. *Life Science* 65:2167-74.

Giannoudis, P.V., Smith, R.M., Banks, R.E., Windsor, A.C., Dickson, R.A., Guillou, P.J. (1998). Stimulation of inflammatory markers after blunt trauma. *The British Journal of Surgery* 85:986-990.

Goodyear, L.J., Chang, P.Y., Sherwood, D.J., Durfesne, S.D., Moller, D.E. (1996). Effects of exercise and insulin on mitogen-activated protein kinase signaling patways in rat skeletal muscle. *American Journal of Physiology* 271:E403-8.

Goto, M., Katayama, K.I, Shirakawa, F, Tanaka, I. (1999). Involement of NF-kB p50/p65 heterodimer in activation of the upstream enhancer element. *Cytokine* 11:16-28.

Hack, C.E., Aarden, L.A., Thijs L.G. (1997). Role of cytokines in sepsis. *Advanced Immunology* 66:101-195.

Hayashi, T., Hirshman, M.F., Dufresne, S.D., Goodyear, L.J. (1999). Skeletal muscle contractile activity in vitro stimulates mitogen-activated protein kinase signaling. *American Journal of Physiology* 277:C701-C707.

Hellsten, Y., Frandsen, U. (1997). Adenosine formation in contracting primary rat skeletal muscle cells and endothelial cells in culture. *Journal of Physiology* (Lond.) 504:695-704.

Hill, C.S., Treisman, R. (1995). Transcriptional regulation by extracellular signals: mechanisms and specificity. *Cell* 80:199-211.

Himeno, E., Nishino, K., Nanri, H., Okazaki, T., Komatsu, T., Ikeda, M. (2001). Evaluation of the effects of exercise and a mild hypocaloric diet on cardiovascular risk factors in obese subjects. *Journal of Uoeh* 23:1-12.

Hjeltnes, N., Galuska, D., Bjornholm, M., Aksnes, A.K., Lannem, A., Zierath, J.R., Wallberg-Henriksson, H. (1998). Exercise-induced overexpression of key regulatory proteins involved in glucose uptake and metabolism in tetraplegic persons: molecular mechanism for improved glucose homeostasis. *The FASEB Journal* 12:1701-1712.

Hong, H., Johnson, P. (1995). Antioxidant enzyme activities and lipid peroxidation levels in exercised and hypertensive rat tissues. *International Journal of Biochemical Cellular Biology* 27:923-931.

Hughes, V.A., Fiatarone, M.A., Fielding, R.A., Kahn, B.B., Ferrara, C.M., Shepherd, P.R., Fisher, E.C., Wolfe, R.R., Elahi, D., Evans, W.J. (1993). Exercise increases muscle GLUT4-levels and insulin action in subjects with impaired glucose tolerance. *American Journal of Physiology* 264:E855-E862.

Huh, J.I., Baek, B.S., Kim, H.J., Kim, J.W., Im, Y.K., Shim, K.H., Kim, Y.J., Baek, Y.H., Chung, H.Y. (1999). Upregulation of endothelial renal nitric oxide synthase by exercise. *Korean Journal of Gerontology* 9:45-49.

Jackson, M.J., Edwards, R.H.T., Symons, M.C.R. (1985). Electron spin resonance studies of intact mammalian skeletal muscle. *Biochimica et Biophysica Acta* 847:185-190.

Jacobs, I. (1986). Blood lactate. Implications for training and sports performance. *Sport Medicine* 3:10-25.

Janssens. S.P., Shimouchi., A., Quertermous, T., Block, D.B., Block, K.D. (1992). cloning and expression of a cDNA encoding human endothelium-dervied relaxing factor/nitric oxide synthase. *The Journal of Biological Chemistry* 267:14519-14522.

Jenkins, R.R. (1988). Free radical chemistry: Regulationship to exercise. *Sport Medicine* 5:156-170.

Jenkins, R.R., Friendland, R., Howald, H. (1984). The relationship of oxygen uptake to superoxide dismutase and catalase activity in human skeletal muscle. *International Journal of Sports Medicine* 5:11-14.

Ji, L.L., Stratman, F.W., Lardy, H.A. (1988). Antioxidant enzyme systems in rat liver and skeletal muscle. *Archives of Biochemistry and Biophysics* 263:150-160.

Ji, L.L. (1992). Antioxidant enzyme response to exercise and aging. *Medicine Science in Sports and Exercise* 25:225-231.

Ji, L.L., Fu, R.G. (1992). Responses of glutathione system and antioxidant enzymes to exhaustive exercise and hydroperoxide. *Journal of Applied Physiology* 72:549-554.

Ji, L.L., Fu, R.G., Mitchell, E. (1992). Glutathione and antioxidant enzyme in skeletal muscle: Effect of fiber type and exercise intensity. *Journal of Applied Physiology* 73:1854-1859.

Ji L.L, Bejma, J. (2000). Free radical generation and oxidative stress with aging and execise: differential effects in the myocardium and liver. *Acta physiologica Scandinavica* 169:343-51.

Jonsdottir, I.H. (2000). Special feature for the Olympics: effects of exercise on the immune system: neuropeptides and their interaction with exercise and immune function. *Immunology and Cell Biology* 78:562-70.

Jonsdottir, I.H., Hoffmann, P. (2000). The significance of intensity and duration of exercise on natural immunity in rats. *Medicine Science in Sports and Exercise* 32:1908-12.

Juto, J.E, Lundberg, C. (1985). Nasal mucosa reaction, catecholamines and lactate during physical exercise. *Acta Oto-laryngologica* 98:533-42.

Kaltschmidt, B., Uherek, M., Volk, B., Baeuerle, P.A., Kaltschmidt, C. (1997). Transcription factor NF κB is activated in primary neurons by amyloid _ peptides and in neurons surrounding early plaques from patients with Alzheimer disease. *Proceedings of the National Academy Science USA* 94: 2642-47.

Kane, D.W., Tesauro, T., Koizumi, T., Gupta., R., Newman, J.H. (1994). Exercise-induced pulmonary vasoconstriction during combined blockade of nitric oxide synthase-adrenergic receptors. *Journal of Clinical Investigation* 93:677-683.

Kanter, M.M., Nolte, L.A., Holloszy, J.O. (1993). Effect of an antioxidant vitamin mixture on lipid peroxidation at rest and postexercise. *Journal of Applied Physiology.* 74:965-969.

Kaufmann, S.H. (1990) Heat shock proteins and the immune response. *Immunology Today* 11:129-136.

Kim, J.D., Yu, B.P., McCarter, R.J., Lee, S.Y., Herlihy, J.T. (1996). Exercise and diet modulate cardiac lipid peroxidation and antioxidant defenses. *Free Radical Biology and Medicine* 20:83-88.

Kjellmer, I. (1964). The effect of exercise on the vascular bed of skeletal muscle. *Acta Physiologica Scandinavica* 62:18-30.

Klein-Nulend, J., Helfrich, M.H., Sterck, J.G., MacPherson, H., Joldersma, M., Ralston S.H., Semeins, C.M., Burger, E.H. (1998). Nitric oxide response to shear stress by human bone cell cultures is endothelial nitric oxide synthase dependent. *Biochemical and Biophysical Research Communications* 250:108-14.

Koller-Strametz, J., Matulla, B., Wolzt, M., Muller, M. (1998). Role of nitric oxide in execise-induced vasodilation in man. *Life Science* 62: 1035-1042.

Kondo, H., Itokawa, Y. (1994). In Exercise and Oxygen Toxicity (Sen, C.K., Packer, L., Hanninen, O., Eds.), *Elsevier Science*, Amsterdam 319-342.

Kraniou, Y., Cameron-Smith, D., Misso, M., Collier, G., Hargeaves, M. (2000). Effects of exercise on GLUT4 and glycogenin gene expression in human skeletal muscle. *Journal of Applied Physiology* 88:794-796.

Krook, A., Widegren, U., Jiang, X.J., Henriksson, J., Wallberg-Henriksson, H., Alessi, D., Zierath, J.R. (2000). Effects of exercise on mitogen-and stress-activated kinase signal transduction in human skeletal muscle. American Journal of Physiology. Regulatory Integrative Comparative. *Physiology* 279: R1716-R1721.

Kumar, C.T., Reddy, V.K., Prasad, M., Thyagaraju, K., Reddanna, P. (1992). Dietary supplementation of vitamin E protects heart tissue from exercise-induced oxidative stress. *Molecular and Cellular Biochemistry* 111:109-115.

Kwon, H.J. (2000). Gene Expression of Proinflammatory Proteins and NF-κB Activation in the Aging Process. M.S. thesis, Pusan National University, Pusan, Korea.

Lapenna, D., De Gioia, S., Ciofani, G., Mezzetti, A., Consoli, A., Di Ilio, C., Cuccurullo, F. (1994). Hypochlorous acid-induced zinc release from thiolate bonds: a potential protective mechanism towards biomolecules oxidant damage during inflammation. *Free radical Biology and Medicine* 20:165-70.

Laughlin, M.H., Armstrong, R.B. (1982). Muscular blood flow distribution patterns as a function of running speed in rats. *American Journal of Physiology* 243:H269-306.

Lew, H., Pyke, S., Quintanilha, A. (1985). Changes in the glutathione status of plasma, liver and muscle following exhaustive exercise in rats. *REBS Letter* 185:262-266.

Locke, M, Noble, E.G, Atkinson, B.G. (1990). Exercising mammals synthesize stress proteins. American Journal of Physiology. *Cell Physiology* 258: C723-C729.

Marietta, M.A. 1993. Nitric oxide synthase structure and mechanism. *Journal of Biological Chemistry* 268:12231-12234.

Marietta, M.A. (1994). Nitric oxide synthase : aspect concerning structure and catalysis. *Cell* 78:927-930.

Maroun, M.J., Mehata, S., Turcotte,R., Cosio, M.G., Hussain, S.N. (1995). Effects of physical conditioning on endogenous nitric oxide output during exercise. *Journal of Applied Physiology* 79:1219-25.

Marsden, P.A., Heng, H.H.Q., Scherer, S.W., Stewart, R.J, Hall, A.V., Shi, X.M., Tsui,L.C., Schappert, K.T. (1993). Structure and chromosomal localization of the human constitutive endothelial nitric oxide synthase gene. *Journal of Biological Chemistry* 268:17478-17488.

Mattson, M.P. (1997). Cellular actions of beta-amyloid precursor protein and its soluble and fibrillogenic derivatives. *Physiology Review* 77:1081-1132.

Mattson, M.P. (2000). Apoptosisin neurodegenerative disorders, *Nature Review*. Molecular Cell Biology (In press).

Mattson, M.P., Laferla, F.M., Chan, S.L., Leissring, M.A., Shepel, P.N., Geiger, J.D. (2000). Calcium singnaling in the ER : its role in neuronal plasticity and neurodegenerative disorders. *Trends in Neuroscience* 23:222-229.

McDonald, L.J., Murad, F. (1996). Nitric oxide and cyclic GMP signaling. *Proceedings of the Society for Experimental Biology and Medicine* 211:1-6.

McGeer, P.L., McGeer, E.G. (1999). Inflammation of the brain in Azheimer's Disease: implication for therapy. *Journal of Leukocyte Biology* 65:409-15.

Meydani, M., Evans, W.J. (1993). Free radicals, exercise, and aging. In: Yu, B.P. ed. Free Radicals in Aging. Boca Raton, FL: *CRC Press*: 183-204.

Miyahara, K., Kawamoto,T., Sase, K., Yui, Y. (1994). Cloning and structure characterization of th human endothelial nitric oxide synthase gene. *FEBS letters* 94:719-726.

Mosser, D.D., Duchaine J., Massie, B. (1993). The DNA-binding activity of the human heat shock transcription factor is regulated in vivo by hsp70. *Molecular and Cellular Biology* 13:5427-5438.

Musch, T.I., Terrell, J.A. (1992). Skeletal muscle blood flow abnormalities in rats with chronic myocardial infarction:rest and exercise. *American Journal of Physiology.* 262:H411-H419.

Nathan, C. (1992). Nitric oxide as a secretory product of mammalian cells. *The FASEB Journal* 6:3051-3064.

Nathan, C., Xie, G. (1994). Nitric oxide synthase : role, tills, and controls. *Cell* 78:915-918.

Nehlsen-Cannarella, S.L., Fagoaga, O.R., Nieman, D.C., Henson, D.A., Butterworth, D.E., Schmitt, R.L., Bailey, E.M., Warren, B.J., Utter, A., Davis, J.M. (1997). Carbohydrate and the cytokine response to 2.5h of running. *Journal of Applied Physiology* 82:1662-1667.

Nieman, D.C. (1997). Immune response to heavy exertion. *Journal of Applied Physiology* 82:1385-1394.

Niess, A.M., Passek, F., Lorenz, I., Schneider, E.M., Dickhuth, H-H., Northoff, H., Fehrenbach, E. (1999). Expression of the antioxidant stress protein heme oxygenase-1 (HO-1) in human leukocytes. *Free Radical Biology and Medicine* 26:184-192.

Ninchida, K.,Harrison,D.G., Navas, J.P., Fisher,A.A., Dockery, S.P., Uematsu, M., Nerem, R.M., Alexander, R.W.E., Murphy,T.G. (1992). Molecular cloning and Characterization of constitutive bovine aortic endothelia cell nitric oxide synthase. *Journal of Clinical Investigation* 90:2092-2096.

Ostrowski, K., Hermann, C., Bangash, A., Schjerling, P., Nielsen, J.N., Pedersen, B.K. (1998b). Atrauma-like elevation of plasma cytokines in humans in response to treadmill running. *Journal of Physiology* (Lond) 513:889-894.

Ostrowski, K., Rohde, T., Zacho, M., Asp, S., Pedersen, B.K. (1998a). Evidence that interlukin-6 is produced in human skeletal muscle during prolonged running. *Journal of Physiology* (Lond) 508:949-953.

Ostrowski, K., Rohde, T., Zacho, M., Asp, S., Pedersen, B.K. (1999). pro-and anti-inflammtory cyto kinet interlukin-6 is produced in human skeletal muscle during prolonged running. *Journal of Physiology* (Lond) 508:949-953.

Overley, L.W. (1998). Free radical and diabetes. *Free Radical Biology and Medicine* 5:113-24.

Papadaki, M., Eskin, S.G., Ruef, J., Runge, M.S., McIntire L.V. (1999). Fluid Shear stress as a regulator of gene expression in vascular cells: possible correlation with diabetic abnormalities. *Diabetes Research and Clinical Practice* 45:89-99.

Pedersen, B.K., Ostrowski, K., Rohde, T., Bruunsgaard, H. (1998). The cytokine response to strenuous exercise. *Canadian Journal of Physiology and Pharmacology* 76:505-511.

Penkowa, M., Giralt, M., Carrasco, J., Hadberg, H., Hidalgo, J. (2000). Impaired inflammatory response and increased oxidative stress and neurodegeneration after brain injury in interleukin-6-deficient mice. *Glia* 32:271-85.

Pollock, J.S., Fostrmann, U., Mitchell, J.A., Warmer, T.D., Schmidt, H., Nakang, M., Murad, F. (1991). Purification and characterization of particulate EDRF synthase from cultured and native bovine aortic endotheial cells. *National Academy Science USA* 88:10480-10484.

Powers, S.K., Ji, L.L., Leeuwenburgh, C. (1999). Exercise training-induced alterations in skeletal muscle antioxidant capacity: a brief review. *Medicine Science in Sports and Exercise* 31:987-997.

Powers, S.K., Lawler, J., Criswell, D., Lieu, F.K., Martin, D. (1992). Aging and respirator muscle metabolic plasticity: effects of endurance training. *Journal of Applied Physiology* 72:1068-1073.

Radak, Z., Zsano, K., Inoue, M., Kizaki, T., Oh-ishi, S., Suzuki, K., Taniquchi, N., Ohno, H. (1995). Superoxide dismutase derivatives reduces oxidative damage in skeletal muscle of rats during exhaustive exercise. *Journal of Applied Physiology* 79:129-135.

Reid, M.B. (1998). Role of nitric oxide in skeletal muscle: synthesis, distribution and functional importance. *Acta Physiologica Scandinavica* 162:401-409.

Reid, M.B., Haack, K.E., Francheck, K.M., Valberg, P.A., Kobzik, L., West, M.S. (1992). Reactive oxygen in skeletal muscle I. Intracellular oxidant kinetics and fatique in vitro. *Journal of Applied Physiology* 73:1797-1804.

Ren, J.M., Semenkovich, C.F., Gulve, E.A., Gao, J., Holloszy, J.O. (1994). Exercise induces rapid increases in GLUT4 expression, glucose transport capacity, and insulin-stimulated glycogen storage in muscle. *Journal of Biological Chemistry* 269:14396-14401.

Reznick, A.Z., Witt, E., Matsumot, M., Packer, L. (1992). Vitamin E inhibits protein oxidation in skeletal muscle of resting and exercising rats. *Biochemical and Biophysical Research Communications* 189:801-806.

River, A., Pene, J., Chanez, P., Anselme, F., Caillaud, C., Prefaut C., Godard, P., Bousquet, J. (1994). Release of cytokines by blood monocytes during strenuous exercise. *International Journal of Sports Medicine* 15:192-198.

Rodgers, M.A., Yamamoto, C., King, D.S., Hagberg, J.M., Ehsani, A.A., Holloszy, J.O. (1988). Improvement in glucose tolerance after 1 wk of exercise in patients with mild NIDDM. *Diabetes Care* 11:613-618.

Rufahl, R.H., Nanjappan, P.G., Woodard, R.W., Marietta, M.A. (1992). Mechanistic probes of N-hydroxylation of L-arginine by the inducible nitric oxide syntase from murine macrophage. *Biochemistry* 31:6822-6828.

Ryder, J.W., Fahlman, R., Wallberg-Henriksson, H., Alessi, D.R., Krook, A., Zierath, J.R. (2000). Effect of contraction on mitogen-activated protein kianse signal transduction in skeletal muscle: involvement of the mitogen- and stress-activated protein kinase 1. *Journal of Biological Chemistry* 275:1457-1462.

Sagan, L.A. (1989). On radiation, paradigms, and hormesis. *Science* 245:574,621.

Sawada, M., Sester, U., Carlson, J.C. (1992). Superoxide radical formation and associated biochemical alterations in the plasma membrane of brain, heart and liver during the lifetime of the rat. *Journal of Cell Biochemistry* 48:296-304.

Seger, R., Krebs, E.G. (1995). The MAPK signaling cascade. *The FASEB Journal* 9:726-735.

Sen, C.K. (1998). Redox signaling and the emerging therapeutic potential of thiol antioxidants. *Biochemical Pharmacology* 55:1747-1758.

Sen, C.K. (1995). Oxidants and antioxidants in exercise. *Journal of Applied Physiology* 79:675-686.

Sen, C.K., Hanninen, O. (1994). Physiological antioxidants. In: Sen, C.K., Packer, L., Hanninen, O. (eds). *Exercise and Oxygen Toxicity.* Elsevier Science Publishers, Amsterdam p89-126.

Sen, C.K., Khanna, S., Reznick, A.Z., Roy, S., Packer, L. (1997). Glutathione regulation of tumor necrosis factor-a-induced NF-kB activation in skeletal muscle-derived L6 cells. *Biochemical and Biophysical Research Communications* 237:645-649.

Sen, C.K., Khanna, S., Reznick, A.Z., Roy, S., Packer, L. (1997). Glutathione regulation of tumor necrosis factor-alpha-induced NF-kappa B activation in skeletal muscle-derived L6 cells. *Biochemical and Biophysical Research Communications* 237:645-649.

Sen, C.K., Packer, L. (1996). Antioxidant and redox regulation of gene transcription. *The Journal Faseb* 10:709-720.

Sessa, W.C., Harrision, J.K., Barber, C.M., Zeng, D., Durieux, M.E., D`Angelo, D.D., Lynch, K.R., Peach, M.J. (1992). Molecular cloning and expression of a cDNA encoding human endothelium cell nitric oxide synthase. *Journal of Biological Chemistry* 267:15274-15276.

Sessa, W.C., Pritchard, K., Seyedi, N., Wang, J., Hintze, T.H. (1994). Chronic exercise in dogs increase coronary vascular nitric oxide production and endothelial cell nitric oxide synthase gene expression. *Circulation Research* 74:349-353.

Shinogi M, Sakaridani, M, Yokoyama, I. (1999). Metallothionein induction in rat liver by dietary restriction or exercise and reduction of exercise-induced hepatic lipid peroxidation. *Biological Pharmacology Bulletin* 22:132-6.

Shinoki, N., Kawasaki, T., Minamino, N., Okahara, K., Ogawa, A., Ariyoshi, H., Sakon,M., Kambayashi, J., Kangawa, K., Monden, M. (1998). Shear stress down-regulates gene transcription and production of adrenomedullin in human aortic endothelial cells. *Journal of Cell Biochemistry* 71:109-15.

Stadman, E.R. (1990). Metal ion-catalyzed oxidation of protein: Biochemical mechanism and biological consequences. *Free Radical Biology and Medicine* 9:315-326.

Stebbing, A. (1982). Hormesis – the stimulation of growth by low levels of inhibitors. *Science Total Enviroment* 22:213-234.

Stebbins, C.L., Carretero, O.A., Mindroiu, t., Longhurst, J.C. (1990). Bradykinin release from contracting skeletal muscle of the cat. *Journal of Applied Physiology* 69:1225-1230.

Stuehr, D.J., Kwon N.S., Nathan, C.F., Griffith, O.W., Feldman, P.L., Wiseman, J. (1991). N-hydoxy-L-arginine is and intermedidate in the biosynthesis of nitric oxide from L-arginine. *Journal of Biology Chemistry* 266:6259-6263.

Sun, A.Y., Chen, Y.M. (1998). Oxidative stress and neurodegenerative disorders. *Journal of Biomedicine Science* 5:401-414.

Tan, S.Y., Chan, W.B., Cheng, W.C., Hagarty, A., Lim, K.T., Quaife, R. (2000). Rapid prenatal diagnosis of chromosome abnormalities. *Singapore Medicine* 41:493-7.

Tanaka, C., Kamata, H., Takeshita, H., Yagisawa, H., Hirata, H. (1997). Redox regulation of lipopolysaccharide (LPS)-induced interleukin-8 (IL-8) gene expression mediated by NF kappa B and AP-1 in human astrocytoma U373 cells. *Biochemical and Biophysical Research Communications* 232:568-73.

Tilg, H., Dinarello, C.A., Mier, J.W. (1997). IL-6 and APPs : anti-inflammatory and immunosuppressive mediators. *Immunology Today* 18:428-432.

Tilg, H., Trehu, E., Atkins, M.B., Dinarello, C.A., Mier, J. (1994). Interlukin-6 (IL-6) as and anti-inflammatory cytokine: induction of circulating IL-1 receptor antagonist and soluble tumor necrosis factor receptor. *Blood* 83: 113-118.

Tomas, T., Phodin , J.A., Sutton, E.T., Bryant, M.W., Price, J.M (1999). Estrogen protects peripheral and cerebral blood vessels from toxicity of Alzheimer peptide amyloid-beta and inflammatory reaction. *Journal of Submicroscipic Cytologic Pathology* 31:571-79.

Tso, J.Y., Aoki, N., Lefer, D., Johnson, G., Lefer, A. (1990). Time course of endothelial dysfunction and myocaridial injury during myocardial ischemia and reperfusion in the cat. *Circulation* 80:1402-1412.

Uematsu, M., Ohara, Y., Navas, J.P., Nishidad, K., Murphy, T.J, Alexander R.W., Nerem, R.M., Harrison, D.G. (1995). Regulation of endotherial cell nitric oxide synthase mRNA expression by shera stress. *American Journal of Physiology* 269: c1371-c1378.

Vina, J., Gimeno, A., Sastre, J., Desco, C., Asensi, M., Pallardo, F.V., Cuesta, A., Ferrero, J.A., Terada, L.S. Repine, J.E. (2000). Mechanism of free radical production in allopurinol. *IUBMB Life* 49:539-544.

Wallberg-Henriksson, H. (1986). Repeated exercise regulates glucose transport capacity in skeletal muscle. *Acta Physiologica Scandinavica* 127:39-43.

Weinstock, C., Konig, D., Harnischmacher, R., Keul, J., Berg, A., Northoff, H. (1997). Effect of exhaustive exercise stress on the cytokines response. *Medicine Science in Sports and Exercise* 29:345-354.

Whicher, J., Biasucci, L., Firal N. (1999). Inflammation , the acute phase response and atherosclerosis. *Clinical Chemistry and Laboratory Medicine* 5:495-503.

Widegren, U., Jiang, X.J., Krook, A., Chibalin, A.V., Bjornholm, M., Tally, M., Roth, R.A., Henriksson, J., Wallberg-Henriksson, H., Zierath, J.R. (1998). Divergent effects of exercise on metabolic and mitogenic signaling pathways in human skeletal muscle. *The FASEB Journal* 12:1379-1389.

Wiesinger, G.F., Quittan, M., Aringer, A., Seeber, B Volc-Platzer, Smolen Graninger, J. (1998). Improvement of physical fitness and muscle strength in Polymyositis/Dermato-myositis patients by a training programme. *British Journal of Rheumatology* 37:196-200.

Witt, E., Reznick, A.Z., Viguie, C.A., Sarke-Reed, P., Packer, L. (1992). Exercise, oxidative damage and effects of antioxidant manipulation. *The Journal of Nutrition* 122:766-773.

Xing, Z., Gauldie, J., Cox, G., Baumann, H., Jordana, M., Lei, X.F., Achong, M.K. (1998). IL-6 is and anti-inflammatory cytokine required for controlling local or systemic acute inflammatory responses. *Journal of Clinical Investigation* 101:311-320.

Yan, Z.Q., Sirsjo, A., Bochaton-Piallat, M.L., Gabbiani, G., Hansson, G.K. (1999). Augmented expression of inducible NO synthase in vascular smooth muscle cells during aging is associated with enhanced NF-kappaB activation. *Arteriosclerosis, Thrombosis, and Vascular Biology* 19:2854.

Yoshio, T., Tomita, K., Homma, M.K., Nonoguchi, H., Yang, T., Yamada, T., Yuasa, Y., Krebs, E.G., Sasaki, S., Marumo, F. (1995). Sequential activation of Raf-1 kinase, mitogen-activated protein (MAP) kinase, and S6 kinase by hyperosmolality in renal cells. *Journal of Biological Chemistry* 269:31296-31301.

Yoshizumi, M., Perrella, M.A.,Burnett, J.C., J.R., Lee, M.E. (1993). Tumor necrosis factor downregulates an endothelial nitric oxide syntase mRNA by shortening its half-life. *Circulation Research* 73:205-209.

Yu, B.P., Masoro, E.J., McMahan, C.A. (1985). Nutritional influences on aging Fischer 344-rat.I. Physical, metabolic, and longevity characteristics. *Journal of Gerontology* 40:657-70.

Yu, B.P. (1994). Cellular defenses against damage from reactive oxygen species. *Physiology Review* 74:139-162.

Yu, B.P., Chung, H.Y. (2001). Stress resistance of calorie restrication for longevity. *Annals of NewYork Academy of Science* 928:39-47.

Zerba, E., Komorowski, T.E., Faukner, J.A. (1990). Free radical injury to skeletal muscles of young, adult and old mice. *American Journal of Physiology* 258:C429-C435.

Zhao, G., Zhang, X., Xu X., Ochoa, M., Hintze, T.H. (1997). Short-term exercise training enhances reflex cholinergic nitric oxide–dependent coronary vasodilation in conscious dogs. *Circulation Research* 80:868-876.

Zou, A.P. (1998). Protective effect of angiotensin II-induced increase in nitric oxide in the renal nedullary circulation. *Hypertension* 31:271-276.

Exercise, Oxidative Stress and Muscle Diseases

M. J. JACKSON[1], D. PATTWELL[1] AND A. MCARDLE[1]

[1]Department of Medicine, University of Liverpool, UK

Correspondence to:

M. J. Jackson, MD. & Ph.D.
Department of Medicine
University of Liverpool
Liverpool
L69 3GA, U.K.

Summary

The beneficial effects of exercise have been well documented, but strenuous or unaccustomed exercise can lead to damage to skeletal muscle. Much data now indicate that contracting skeletal muscle produces increased amounts of reactive oxygen and nitrogen species (ROS) during contractile activity. These species have been implicated in the pathogenesis of exercise-induced muscle damage, ageing-related muscle dysfunction and in some muscle diseases although firm evidence in support of this is missing. Recent data also indicate that ROS can play a major role in modulating changes in gene expression in muscle further supporting a key role for these species in maintenance of muscle integrity.

1   Introduction

1.1   Health benefits of exercise

Participation in regular exercise decreases morbidity and appears to be associated with a reduced risk of certain cancers and cardiovascular disorders (Powers and Howley, 1994). Nevertheless unaccustomed or excessive exercise is recognised to have short term deleterious effects on skeletal muscle viability and to result in muscle pain and discomfort (Newham et al., 1988). The possibility that these apparent negative effects of exercise can play a role in the onset or propagation of muscle degeneration in certain disease states or ageing-related muscle dysfunction is receiving increasing attention. This interest has been increased by the observation that exercise is associated with an increased generation of reactive oxygen species, substances that have been implicated in the pathogenesis of both Duchenne muscular dystrophy and ageing-related muscle dysfunction. This review will examine the evidence that skeletal muscle is a source for generation of reactive oxygen species during exercise and consider whether this generation plays a role in muscle degeneration in muscular dystrophy and ageing-related muscle dysfunction.

1.2 Contracting skeletal muscle is a source of reactive oxygen species during exercise

Tappel and co-workers appear to have been the first to suggest that exercise in humans is associated with increased oxygen free radical generation (Dillard et al., 1978). Studies using a variety of different approaches have supported this possibility (e.g see Davies et al., 1982; Jackson et al., 1985) and it has been suggested that skeletal muscle is a likely source of reactive oxygen species since the oxygen uptake by skeletal muscle may increase by two orders of magnitude during some forms of contraction. It is now clear that in addition to generation of reactive oxygen species (ROS) within the tissues, a number of reactive oxygen species are released into the muscle extracellular space during contractile activity. Reid et al. (1992) reported that strips of diaphragm released increased amounts of superoxide anion during stimulated contractile activity and we have recently demonstrated that this anion is released from skeletal muscle cells *per se* rather than other cell types within the tissue during contraction (McArdle et al., 2001). Skeletal muscle also releases nitric oxide (NO) to the extracellular medium during contraction (Balon and Nadler, 1996), most probably deriving from a plasma membrane-located type I (neuronal-type) nitric oxide synthase (nNOS, Hirschfield et al., 2000; Reid, 1996). An increase in extracellular hydroxyl radicals has also been observed during muscle contractile activity in vivo (O'Neill et al., 1996). The formation of these species appears to occur within the extracellular space by iron-catalysed breakdown of hydrogen peroxide released from the skeletal muscle (O'Neill et al., 1996).

1.3 Sub-cellular sources for generation of reactive oxygen species in contracting skeletal muscle

Mitochondria are considered by many authors to be the primary source of the superoxide generation in skeletal muscle (e.g. Davies et al., 1982; Reid et al., 1992) and electron spin resonance studies have demonstrated an increase in mitochondrial ubisemiquinone (Jackson et al., 1985; Jackson and Johnson, 1989) that may be a source of mitochondrial superoxide generation during contraction. However this cannot explain the increased release of extracellular superoxide anions from contracting muscle (Reid et al., 1992; McArdle et al., 2001). Superoxide anions are charged and reactive and diffusion from the mitochondria across both mitochondrial and plasma membranes to the extracellular space seems unlikely. Mitochondrial superoxide is also rapidly converted by manganese superoxide dismutase (MnSOD) to hydrogen peroxide which is capable of diffusion from the muscle cells and may provide a potential substrate for the iron-catalysed generation of extracellular hydroxyl radicals (O'Neill et al., 1996). Various alternative sources for the generation of extracellular superoxide have been suggested (McArdle et al., 2001).

A schematic diagram of the different reactive oxygen species generated by skeletal muscle and their likely sources of generation is shown in Figure 1.

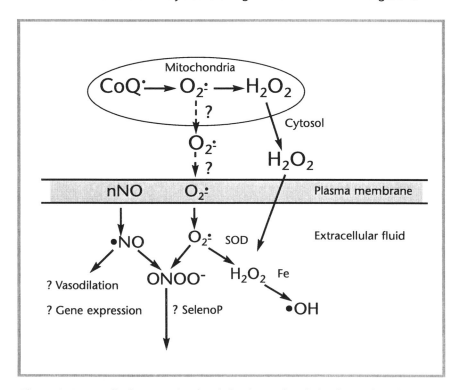

Figure 1. *Free radical generation by skeletal muscle. Skeletal muscle is known to generate superoxide from mitochondria and superoxide, hydroxyl radicals and nitric oxide are known to be released to the extracellular space during muscle contraction. Although mitochondrial generation of superoxide is likely to be quantitatively the major source of oxidants in contracting skeletal muscle, it appears unlikely that the superoxide generated within mitochondria can diffuse across both mitochondrial and plasma membranes to provide the superoxide detected in the extracellular space (Reid et al, 1992; McArdle et al, 2001). This appears to be generated from an undefined plasma membrane-located source (McArdle et al, 2001). Hydrogen peroxide generated by the action of MnSOD on superoxide within mitochondria is capable of diffusion and may provide a substrate for the iron-dependant generation of hydroxyl radicals in the extracellular fluid (O'Neill et al, 1996). Neuronal nitric oxide synthase (nNOS) is associated with a1-syntrophin in the complex of dystrophin-associated proteins in the muscle plasma membrane and appears to be the major source of NO released by skeletal muscle (Hirschfield et al, 2000).*

1.4 Actions of reactive oxygen species generated by contracting skeletal muscle

Despite much speculation concerning the possibility that the reactive oxygen species generated during contractile activity are involved in the pathogenesis of exercise-induced skeletal muscle damage or fatigue, there is little firm evidence in support of this. A period of unaccustomed or excessive contractile activity may lead to an increase in indicators of lipid, DNA or protein oxidation in skeletal muscle, but there is little evidence that repeated exposure of normal skeletal muscle to the various oxidants generated during contractile activity leads to sustained damage to the tissue (Jackson, 1998 for a review).

1.5 Contraction induces specific adaptive responses to prevent oxidative damage to skeletal muscle

Most published studies indicate that muscle cells adapt to contraction by upregulation of the activity of "antioxidant" enzymes to reduce the risk of damage to the tissue by any subsequent increases in free radical activity. In animals, an acute bout of exercise (Ji, 1993; McArdle et al., 2001) or longer term exercise training (Higuchi et al. 1985; Ji, 1993) increase the activities of superoxide dismutase, catalase and glutathione peroxidase in muscle and comparable data have been reported from studies in humans (Jenkins et al., 1984; Robertson et al., 1991, Khassaf et al., 2001). In addition other cytoprotective proteins, such as the heat shock proteins (HSPs), particularly HSP60, 70 and 25, are important components of the cellular protective response against reactive oxygen species and recent data indicate that an increase in the muscle content of HSPs occurs following exercise in rats (Salo et al., 1991; Kelly et al., 1996; Hernando and Manso, 1997), contractile activity of muscle in mice (McArdle et al., 2001) or exercise in man (Khassaf et al., 2001).

Reactive oxygen species play an important role in regulating the intracellular redox balance, influencing the activity of several key transcription factors and signalling molecules and leading to modulation of the expression of those genes controlled by these pathways (Ammendola et al., 1995; Stortz and Polla, 1996; Lander et al., 1996). Some of the adaptive changes induced by contractile activity in skeletal muscle appear to be directly mediated by reactive oxygen species. We have demonstrated that the increased muscle HSP content that occurs following an acute period of muscle exercise in man (Khassaf et al., 2001) is attenuated by prior supplementation with vitamin C and other nutritional antioxidants (Jackson et al., 1999; Khassaf et al., 1999). Tidball and colleagues have also reported that changes in muscle protein composition in response to some mechanical stimuli are mediated by NO-induced changes in gene expression (Tidball et al., 1999; Kohl and Tidball, 1999).

In summary therefore it is clear that skeletal muscle generates reactive oxygen species during contractions and that normal muscle cells respond to minimise the risk of damage caused by the increased generation of these oxidants.

2   Muscle Dysfunction and Ageing

2.1   Failure of skeletal muscle function occurs during ageing

Declining muscle strength, muscle wasting and physical frailty are an accepted part of ageing such that by the age of 70 skeletal muscle cross–sectional area is reduced by 25-30% and muscle strength is reduced by 30-40% (Porter et al., 1995). The loss of muscle strength continues to fall by 1-2% per year (Skelton et al., 1994). This deficit has a profound impact on the quality of life of older people. Loss of muscle strength leads to instability, a subsequent increased risk of falls and consequently an increased need for residential care. A large number of healthy older people are at, or near to, functionally important strength-related thresholds and so have lost or are close to losing the ability to carry out everyday tasks (Young and Skelton, 1994). In addition, the age-related decline in muscle bulk and strength contributes to other risk factors in older people, including an increased susceptibility to hypothermia and increased incidence of incontinence.

The structural changes which are responsible for this age-related fall in muscle strength have been well documented (see Porter et al., 1995 for a review). Studies indicate that most healthy older subjects are able to activate their muscle maximally during voluntary contraction (Vandervoort and McComas, 1986). The age-related decline in muscle volume and cross sectional area is due to both a significant decrease in the total number of individual muscle fibres within the muscle bulk and an atrophy of the remaining fibres. This atrophy appears to primarily occur in type II (fast, glycolytic) fibre, the cross sectional area of type I (slow, oxidative) fibres being relatively well maintained (Lexell et al., 1988). The reduction in the proportion of type II fast muscle fibres results in the muscle moving towards the characteristics of type I or slow muscle fibres. Thus a slowing of contraction, rate of force development and so a reduced ability to accelerate the movement of a limb is observed, amplifying the impact of muscle weakness on stability (Larsson et al., 1979; Stanley and Taylor, 1993).

The remaining muscle fibres in muscles of aged mice generate less force per unit cross sectional area than a similar sized young muscle (Brooks and Faulkner, 1988; McBride et al., 1995). Thus, loss of muscle fibres accounted for a proportion of the overall force deficit in muscles of aged mice, but did not account for all of this loss and the force generated per unit cross sectional area was ~25% less than that from muscles of young mice (Faulkner et al., 1990a & b).

2.2 Aged muscle is more susceptible to contraction-induced damage

Although there are no definitive studies of the susceptibility of aged human muscle to contraction-induced damage, several studies have demonstrated that skeletal muscle of aged rodents is more susceptible to contraction-induced damage than that of young animals and also takes longer to recover from damage than young animals (Faulkner 1990a). Contraction-induced skeletal muscle damage may occur whenever muscle is exposed to unaccustomed or excessive periods of exercise, but by far the most damaging form is where the muscle is lengthened during the contraction. Skeletal muscles of aged rodents are significantly more susceptible to this form of contraction–induced damage (McBride et al., 1995; Zerba et al., 1990). In studies from Faulkner's laboratory, the force deficit following a sub-maximal damaging exercise protocol was ~36% in muscles of young mice and ~57% in muscles of old mice (Brooks and Faulkner, 1988; Zerba et al., 1990). This damage also takes considerably longer to repair in old mice such that the muscles from young mice had recovered their ability to generate force by 28 days following the damaging exercise, whereas a significant deficit remained in the muscles of the old mice at 60 days following the exercise.

Work from Faulkner's and our laboratories also indicates that lengthening contraction-induced damage to skeletal muscle is mediated, in part, by reactive oxygen species (Zerba et al., 1990; McArdle et al., 1999). Thus these data are compatible with the possibility that aged skeletal muscle has an increased susceptibility to reactive oxygen species generated by lengthening contractions.

2.3 Ageing is associated with increased oxidative damage to all tissues and reduction in ROS increases longevity in model organisms

Oxidative processes appear to play an important role in the pathogenesis of common ageing-related disorders such as coronary heart disease and a variety of cancers, in addition to a fundamental role in the ageing process (Halliwell and Gutteridge, 1989; Ames et al., 1993; Harman, 1992). All tissues of aged organisms contain accumulated products of oxidative damage to biomolecules such as phospholipid, DNA and proteins (Schoneich, 1999; Nohl, 1993). Most interest has focussed on the role of oxidants derived from mitochondria in this damage. Aged mitochondria contain significant amounts of oxidative damage associated with a marked increase in the number of rearrangements of mitochondrial DNA (Melov et al., 1995). Sohal et al., (1994) suggest that these changes are due to an increase in mitochondrial superoxide and hydrogen peroxide production with increasing age, a hypothesis supported by studies in non-mammalian systems where overexpression of Cu,Zn-superoxide dismutase and catalase caused an extension of life span in *Drosophila melanogaster*

(Orr and Sohal, 1994). This possibility is also supported by the recent description of extended lifespan in C. Elegans treated with a Mn-superoxide dismutase (MnSOD) and catalase mimetic (Melov et al., 2000).

2.4 Oxidative stress, exercise and ageing of skeletal muscle

Aged skeletal muscle and other tissues contain increased levels of oxidative damage to DNA, proteins etc. (Sohal et al., 1994). There is little direct evidence to indicate that this oxidation arises directly from the oxidants generated by contractions. Subjects who regularly participate in exercise throughout life appear to maintain muscle bulk and function better than sedentary cohorts (Grimby, 1995). This apparent discrepancy can be explained if there is a progressive failure to adapt to the oxidative stress of contraction during ageing as we have previously proposed (McArdle and Jackson, 2001).

A failure to adapt to environmental change is characteristic of the ageing process (Driscoll, 1971; Oeschli and Bueckley, 1970) although this has not been well defined at the cellular level. The heat shock response shows characteristic changes with ageing. Ageing results in a 50% reduction in induction of HSPs following thermal stress in rat hepatocytes (Heydani et al., 1994) due to a failure of transcription of the HSP genes (Pahlavani et al., 1995). This appears to related to defective function of heat shock transcription factor-1 (HSF1). Of particular relevance in this area is that an attenuated HSP response occurs in skeletal muscle of aged rodents in comparison with young animals in response to contractile activity (Vasilaki et al., 2002).

In summary therefore data indicate that reactive oxygen species play a fundamental role in the ageing process in all tissues, but whether the reactive oxygen species generated during contractions are involved in skeletal muscle ageing is still unclear.

3 Muscular Dystrophy

3.1 Lack of dystophin leads to Duchenne muscular dystrophy

The genetic defect responsible for Duchenne and Becker muscular dystrophy (DMD and BMD) has been identified (Monaco et al., 1985) and localised to band Xp21 on the human X chromosome. The cloned gene was used to identify the protein product, named dystrophin (Hoffman et al., 1987), which was shown to be absent or greatly diminished (<3%) in muscle from DMD patients (Hoffman et al., 1987).

It has subsequently been shown that dystrophin is absent in three animal models of muscular dystrophy, the mdx mouse, the XMD dog and the dystrophic cat (Hoffman et al., 1987; Cooper et al., 1989; Carpenter et al.,

1989). The elucidation of these animal models has had a dramatic effect on studies of the pathophysiology of Duchenne muscular dystrophy. In particular, the short breeding time, low relative cost and availability of the mdx mouse model has facilitated a large number of recent studies of the potential role of dystrophin in normal muscle and of the means by which a lack of this protein leads to the development of the dystrophic process.

Dystrophin is found in skeletal, cardiac and smooth muscle (Karpati and Carpenter, 1988) and proteins from the small C-terminal transcripts of the same gene are found in other tissues (Chamberlain et al., 1993). Immunohistological staining using antibodies raised against dystrophin located the protein on the cytoplasmic side of the plasma membrane (Watkins et al., 1988; Cullen et al., 1990). Karpati and Carpenter (1988) initially proposed that dystrophin was orientated with its N terminal attached to actin of the cytoskeleton, and the C terminal anchored through the plasma membrane. Various research groups (Ervasti and Campbell, 1991; Yoshida and Ozawa, 1990) have demonstrated that dystrophin is a cytoplasmic protein which exists in association with a large, plasma membrane spanning, oligomeric glycoprotein complex, which is now thought to be attached to the merosin (laminin M) component of the muscle extracellular matrix (Ibraghiminov-Baskrovnaya et al., 1992), although the precise molecular organisation of the glycoprotein-dystrophin complex is unclear (Ervasti and Campbell, 1991; Suzuki et al., 1994). Lack of dystrophin appears to lead to the loss of these associated proteins in mdx mouse and DMD muscle (Ervasti et al., 1990; Ohlendieck and Campbell, 1991). It has been suggested that it may be the loss of one or more of these associated proteins, or the whole complex, that leads to the degeneration seen in dystrophin-deficient muscle since the specific loss of one of the associated glycoproteins in the presence of apparently normal expression and localisation of dystrophin, results in a myopathy similar to DMD (Matsumura et al., 1992; Sewry et al., 1994). Furthermore, data also indicate that patients with congenital muscular dystrophy have a specific reduction in merosin in muscle extracellular matrix (Hayashi et al., 1993), further supporting the idea that defects in various parts of this protein/glycoprotein structure leads to myopathy.

3.2 A role for exercise in the muscle degeneration in muscular dystrophy?

The precise function for dystrophin remains to be elucidated although various theories have been proposed concerning the function of the protein in skeletal muscle. One well characterised theory (the mechanical damage hypothesis) is particularly relevant to understanding the responses of dystrophic muscle to exercise.

Following the identification of the genetic and phenotypic defect responsible for DMD, Karpati and Carpenter (1988) adapted the initial 'Mechanical Damage

Hypothesis' of Edwards et al., (1984) to propose a possible function for dystrophin. Based on the structure and location of dystrophin within the muscle fibres, Karpati and Carpenter (1988) proposed that dystrophin provides mechanical stability to the muscle plasma membrane against the substantial stresses placed on it during normal muscle contraction. This potential role of dystrophin in mechanical stability was supported by experimental work from the same group (Weller et al., 1990). These authors argued that the use of muscles in lengthening contractions was particularly damaging to normal muscle by increasing the mechanical stresses on the muscle fibre (Warren et al., 1993) and that dystrophin-deficient muscle would be more susceptible to this form of damage. Weller et al., (1990) reported an increased susceptibility of anterior tibialis (AT) muscles from 100 day old mdx mice to lengthening contractions 'in vivo'. Recent loss of viability of muscle fibres was assessed by positive staining of individual fibres for IgG. However, mice of the age studied by this group show signs of on-going degeneration and deformed fibres (Cullen and Jaros, 1988; Head et al., 1992). Thus, the increased loss of viability observed with eccentric contractions may have occurred in fibres already compromised by the underlying degenerative process. Head et al. (1992) have shown that between 5 and 40% of fibres in muscles from mdx mice of this age are abnormal and suggest that it is these already compromised fibres that have an increased susceptibility to eccentric contraction-induced damage.

Data examining the effect of eccentric contractions on procion orange exclusion by dystrophic muscle fibres was also provided in the studies of Weller et al. (1990). Petrof et al. (1993) demonstrated that fibres from 90-110 day old mdx mice exhibited an increased susceptibility to contraction-induced sarcolemmal rupture. A specific susceptibility of EDL muscles from adult mdx mice to eccentric activity-induced damage was claimed by Moens et al. (1993), although soleus muscles subjected to eccentric activity and either soleus or EDL muscles subjected to isometric activity displayed force losses and accumulation of procion red comparable with control muscles. However, again the mice studied by both Petrof et al. (1993) and Moens et al. (1993) would have muscles which had undergone previous periods of degeneration and regeneration and the changes may represent a precipitation of loss of viability in already degenerating cells or an increased susceptibility of regenerated but deformed cells to contraction induced damage, rather than a true increased susceptibility of all dystrophin-deficient fibres per se to this form of damage.

Directly contradictory data were presented by Sacco et al. (1992) who studied an alternative measure of damage, the loss of force generation, by muscles from 16-26 week old mdx mice subjected to repetitive eccentric contractile activity 'in vivo'. They observed no significant difference between mdx and age-matched control muscles.

Work by our group (McArdle et al., 1991; 1992) did not support the 'Mechanical Damage Hypothesis' in that we could not demonstrate an increased susceptibility of isolated extensor digitorum longus (EDL) muscles from 40 day old mdx mice to damage caused by both isometric and eccentric activity 'in vitro' in comparison with muscles from control animals. Two alternative indicators of damage to muscle were examined for these studies; the release of intracellular creatine kinase and accumulation of extracellular ^{45}Ca. These results did not appear to be complicated by the presence of regenerating fibres in the mdx muscles since control studies with regenerating muscle in the same system under the same conditions demonstrated a similar susceptibility to contraction-induced damage (McArdle et al., 1994).

Work from other species is also relevant although also inconclusive in indicating the relative susceptibility of dystrophin-deficient muscle to mechanical damage. Studies of the effect of eccentric exercise on patients with DMD do not indicate an increased susceptibility to this form of damage (Jackson et al., 1987) in contrast to the theoretical calculations undertaken by Edwards et al. (1984). However, it is also clear that the XMD dog shows substantial increased susceptibility to exercise-induced muscle damage (Valentine et al., 1989).

It is therefore apparent that there is considerable discrepancy between the results of studies to examine the possibility that dystrophin provides mechanical stability to the muscle plasma membrane during contractile activity.

3.3 Abnormal NOS distribution in dystrophic muscle

A causative link between muscle degeneration in Duchenne muscular dystrophy and damage by reactive oxygen species has been proposed for a considerable period of time (see Jackson et al., 1984), although with elucidation of the underlying defect in DMD there did not appear to be a clear pathogenic rationale for an involvement of reactive oxygen species in the damaging process. DMD muscle contains increased amounts of products of oxidative damage to lipids (Jackson et al., 1984) and some data indicate that this is also true of muscle from the mdx mouse model of the disease (Disatnik et al., 1998), although this is not a universal finding (Foxley et al., 1991). The recent observation that nNOS is linked with dystrophin in skeletal muscle (Bonilla et al., 1988) provides a potential rationale for an involvement of reactive oxygen species in muscle degeneration in DMD muscle. nNOS appears to bind to a1-syntrophin in the complex of dystrophin-associated proteins (Kameye et al., 1999) and a lack of dystrophin in DMD and mdx muscle causes loss of nNOS from the sarcolemma and a diffuse redistribution of the enzyme within the cytoplasm (Chang et al., 1996). Total nNOS activity may also be reduced (Brenman et al., 1995).

A direct effect of this redistribution of nNOS on NO production by dystrophic skeletal muscle does not appear to have been demonstrated, but could conceivably lead to an abberant superoxide production by DMD muscle during contractions (see figure 1) leading to the increased oxidative damage previously reported in dystrophic muscle. Despite this plausible hypothesis, studies with transgenic and knockout animlas do not support a crucial involvement of nNOS in degeneration of dystrophic muscle. Knockout mice lacking nNOS show no evidence of muscle degeneration (Chao et al., 1998) and joint knockout animals lacking both dystrophin and nNOS show the same pattern of degeneration as mice lacking dystrophin alone (Chao et al., 1998)

In summary therefore dystrophic muscle may show some increased sensitivity to contraction-induced damage, but this may be a secondary effect due to the presence of previously damaged fibres. There is also little firm evidence in support of a fundamental role of reactive oxygen species in muscle damage in this disorder.

Acknowledgements

The authors would like to thank the *Wellcome Trust, Research into Ageing, Biotechnology and Biological Sciences Research Council and Mersey Kidney Research* for financial support of their studies.

REFERENCES

Ames BN, Shigenaga MK and Hagan TM (1993). *Proc. Natl. Acad. Sci. USA* 91: 915-922.

Ammendola R, Fiore F, Esposito F, Caserta G, Mesuraca M, Russo T and Cimino F (1995). *FEBS Lett.* 371:209-213.

Balon TW, Nadler JL (1994). *J. Appl. Physiol.* 77:2519-2521.

Bonilla E, Samitt CE, Miranda AF et al. (1988). *Cell* 54:447-452.

Brenman JE, Chao DS, Xia H, Aldape K and Bredt DS (1995). *Cell* 82:743-752.

Brooks SV and Faulkner JA (1988). *J. Physiol.* 404:71-82

Chang WJ, Iannaccone St, Lau KS et al. (1996). *Proc. Natl. Acad. Sci.* USA 93: 9142-9147.

Chao DS, Silvagno F and Bredt DS (1998). *J. Neurochem.* 71:784-789.

Choi AMK and Alam J (1996). *Am. J. Resp. Cell. Mol. Biol.* 15:9-19.

Carpenter JL, Hoffman EP and Romanul FCA (1989). *Am. J. Pathol.* 135:909-919.

Chamberlain JS, Phelps SF, Cox GA, Maichele AJ and Greenwood AD (1993). In: Partridge T ed. *Molecular and cell biology of muscular dystrophy.* London: Chapman and Hall, pp. 167-189.

Cooper BJ, Winand NJ and Stedman H (1988). *Nature* 334:154-156.

Cullen MJ and Jaros E. *Acta Neuropathol.* 1988; 77:69-81.

Cullen MJ, Walsh J, Nicholson LVB and Harris JB (1990). *Proc. R. Soc. Lond.* 240: 197-210.

Davies KJA, Quintanilla AT, Brooks GA and Packer L (1982). *Biochem. Biophys. Res. Comm.* 107:1198-1205.

Dillard CJ, Litov RE, Savin WM, Dumelin EE and Tappel AL (1978). *J. Appl. Physiol.* 45:927-932.

Disatnik MH, Dhawan J, Yu Y, Beal MF, Whirl MM, Franco AA and Rando TA (1998). *J. Neurol. Sci.* 161:77-84.

Driscoll DM (1971). *Int. J. Biometeriol.* 15: 23-29.

Edwards RHT, Jones DA, Newham DA and Chapman SJ (1984). *Lancet i:* 548-551.

Ervasti JM and Campbell KP (1991). *Cell* 66:1121-1131

Ervasti JM, Ohlendieck K, Kahl SD, Gaver MG and Campbell KP (1990). *Nature* 345:315-319.

Evans PJ, Smith C, Mitchinson MJ and Halliwell B (1995). *Free Rad.* Res. 23: 465-469.

Faulkner JA, Brooks SV and Zerba E (1990a). *Ann.Rev Gerontol Geriatr.* 10: 47-66.

Faulkner JA, Brooks SV and Zerba E (1990b). *Hermes (Leuven)* XXI:69-280.

Foxley A., Edwards RH, Jackson MJ (1991). *Biochem. Soz. Trans.* 19:1805.

Grimby G (1995). *J. Gerontol.* 50A:17-22.

Grimby G and Saltin B (1982). *Clin. Physiol.* 3:209-218.

Halliwell, B and Gutteridge JMC (1989). *Free radical biology and medicine.* Oxford University Press.

Harman D (1992). In: Free radicals and ageing. Birkhauser-Verlag, Basel. Pp. 1-10.

Hayashi YK, Engvall E, Arikaea-Hirasawa E et al. (1993). *J. Neurol. Sci.* 119:53-64.

Head SI, Williams DA and Stephenson DG (1992). *Proc. R. Soc. Lond. B.* 248:163-169.

Hempel SL, Buettner GR, O'Malley YQ, Wessels DA and Flaherty DM (1994). *Free Rad. Biol. Med.* 27:146-159.

Hernando R and Manso R (1997). *Eur. J. Biochem.* 243:460-467.

Heydani AR, Takahashi R, Gutsmann A, You S and Richardson A (1994). *Experientia* 50:1092-1098.

Higuchi M, Cartier LJ, Chen M and Holloszy JO (1985). *J. Gerontol.* 40:281-286.

Hirschfield W, Moody Mr, O'Brien W, Gregg AR, Bryan RM Jr. and Reid MB (2000). *Am. J. Physiol.* 278:R95-R100.

Hoffman EP, Brown RH, and Kunkel LM (1987). *Cell* 51:919-928.

Ibraghiminov-Beskrovnaya O, Ervasti JM, Leville CJ, Slaughter CA, Sernett SW and Campbell KP (1992). *Nature* 355:696-702

Jackson MJ, Edwards RHT and Symons MCR (1985). *Biochim. Biophys. Acta* 847, 185-190.

Jackson MJ, Jones DA and Edwards RHT (1984). *Med. Biol.* 62:135-138.

Jackson MJ, Round JM, Newham DJ and Edwards RHT (1987). *Muscle and Nerve* 10:15-21.

Jackson MJ (1998). In: Oxidative stress in skeletal muscle. [A.Z. Reznick, L. Packer, C.K. Sen, J.O. Holloszy, M.J.Jackson Eds.]. Pub. Birkhauser Verlag, Basel (1998) pp. 75-86.

Jackson MJ and Johnson K (1989). In: *CRC Handbook of Biomedicine of Free Radicals and Antioxidants.* Vol III [J. Miguel, A. Quintanilla and H. Weber Eds.] CRC Press. pp 209-213.

Jackson MJ, Khassaf M, Esanu C, Vasilaki A, Brodie DA and McArdle A (1999). *Free Rad. Biol. Med.* 27:S36.

Jenkins RR, Friedland R and Howald H (1984). *Int. J. Sports Med.* 5:11-14.

Ji LL (1993). *Med. Sci. Sports Exercise.* 25:225-231.

Kameye S, Miyagoe Y, Nonaka I et al. (1999). *J. Biol. Chem.* 274:2193-2200.

Karpati G and Carpenter S (1988). In: Sellin LC, Libelius R, Thesleff S eds. *Neuromuscular Junction.* Elsevier Science pp. 429-436.

Kelly DA, Tiidus PM, Houston ME and Noble EG (1996). *J. Appl. Physiol.* 81: 2379-2385.

Khassaf, M., Child RB, McArdle A, Brodie DA, Esanu C and Jackson MJ (2001). *J. Appl. Physiol.* 90:1031-1035.

Khassaf M, McArdle A, Vasilaki A, Esanu C, Brodie DA and Jackson MJ (1999). *Free Rad.. Biol. Med.* 27:S37.

Koh TJ and Tidball JG (1999). *J. Physiol.* 519:189-196.

Lander HM, Milbank AJ and Tauras JM et al. (1996) *Nature* 381:390-381.

Larson L Grimby G and Karlsson J (1979). *J. Appl. Physiol.* 46:451-456.

Lexell J (1993). *Can J. Appl. Physiol.* 18:2-18.

Lexell J, Taylor CC and Sjostrom M. (1988). *J Neurol Sci.* 84:275-294

McArdle A, Edwards RHT and Jackson MJ (1991) *Clin. Sci.* 80:367-371.

McArdle A, Edwards RHT and Jackson MJ (1992). *Clin. Sci.* 82:455-459.

McArdle A, Edwards RHT and Jackson MJ (1994). *J. Appl. Physiol.* 73(3):1274-1278.

McArdle A and Jackson MJ (2000). *J. Anat.* 197:539-541.

McArdle A, van der Meulen J Catapano M, Symons MCR, Faulkner JA and Jackson MJ (1999). *Free Rad. Biol. Med.* 26:1085-1091.

McArdle A, Pattwell D, Vasilaki A, Griffiths RD and MJ Jackson (2001). *Am. J. Physiol.* 280:C621-C627.

McBride TA, Gorin FA and Carlsen RC (1995). *Mech Ageing Dev.* 83:185-200.

Matsumura K, Torne MS, Collin H et al. (1992). *Nature* 359:320-322.

Moens P, Baatsen PHWW and Marechal G (1993). *J. Musc. Res. Cell Motil.* 1993; 14:446-451.

Monaco AP, Bertelson CJ, Middlesworth W et al. (1985). *Nature* 316:842-845.

Melov S, Ravenscroft J, Malik S et al. (2000). *Science* 289:1567-1569.

Newham DJ, Jones DA, Ghosh G and Aurora P (1988). *Clin. Sci.* 74:553-557.

Oeschli FW and Bueckley RW (1970). *Environ. Res.* 3:277-284.

Ohlendieck K and Campbell KP (1991). *J. Cell. Biol.* ; 115(6):1685-1694.

O'Neill CA, Stebbins CL, Bonigut S, Halliwell B and Longhurst JC (1996). *J. Appl. Physiol.* 81:1197-1206.

Orr WC and Sohal RS (1994). *Science* 263:1128-1130.

Pahlavani MA, Harris MD, Moore SA, Weindruch R and Richardson A (1998). *Exptl. Cell Res.* 218:310-318.

Pattwell D, McArdle A, Griffiths RD and Jackson MJ (2001). *Free Rad. Biol. Med.* 30:979-985.

Petrof BJ, Shrager JB, Stedman HH, Kelly AM and Sweeney HL (1993) *Proc. Natl. Acad. Sci. USA.* 99:3710-3714.

Porter MM, Vandervoort AA and Lexell J (1995). *Scand J Med Sci Sports.* 5:129-142

Powers SK and Howley ET (1994). Exercise Physiology. Pub. Madison: Brown and Benchmark.

Reid MB (1996). *News Physiol. Sci.* 11:114-119.

Reid MB, Shoji T, Moody MR and Entman ML (1992). *J. Appl. Physiol.* 75: 1805-1809.

Robertson JD, Maughan RJ, Duthie GG and Morrice PC (1991). *Clin. Sci.* 80: 611-618.

Sacco P, Jones DA, Dick JRT and Vrbova, G (1992). *Clin. Sci.* 1992; 82:227-236.

Salo, DC, Donovan CM and Davies KJA (1992). *Free Rad. Biol. Med.* 11:239-246.

Sewry CA, Sansome A, Matsumura K, Campbell KP and Dubowitz (1994). *Neuromusc. Disord.* 4(2):121-129.

Skelton DA, Greig CA, Davies JM and Young A (1994). *Age Ageing.* 23:371-377.

Sohal RS, Ku HH, Agarwal S, Forster MJ and Lal H (1994a). *Mech. Ageing Dev.* 74:121-133.

Sohal RS, Agarwal S, Candas M, Forster MJ and Lal H (1994b). *Mech. Ageing Dev.* 76:215-224.

Stanley SN and Taylor NAS (1993). *Eur. J. Appl. Physiol.* 66:198-184.

Storz G, and Polla BS (1996). In: Stress inducible cellular responses [U. Feige, RII Morimoto, I Yahara and BS Polla, Eds]. Basel: Birkhauser Verlag. pp 239-254.

Suzuki A, Yoshida M, Hayashi K, Mizuno Y, Hagiwara Y and Ozawa E (1994). *Eur. J. Biochem.* 220:283-292.

Tidball JG, Spencer MJ, Wehling M and Lavergne E (1999). *J. Biol. Chem.* 274: 33155-33160.

Tsuji Y, Ayaki H, Whitman SP, Morrow CS, Torti SV and Torti FM (2000). *Mol. Cell. Biol.* 20:5818-5827.

Valentine BA, Blue JT and Cooper BJ (1989). *Ann. Neurol..* 588.

Vandervoort AA and McComas AJ (1986). *J Appl Physiol.* 61(1):361-7.

Vasilaki A, McArdle A and Jackson MJ (2002). *Muscle and Nerve* 25: 902-905.

Vojtesek B, Dolezalova H, Lauerova L et al. (1995). *Oncogene* 10:389-393.

Warren GL, Hayes DA, Lowe DA, Prior BM and Armstrong, CB (1993). *J. Physiol.* 464:477-489.

Watkins SC, Hoffman EP, Slater HS and Kunkel LM (1988). *Nature* 333:863-866.

Weller B, Karpati G and Carpenter S (1990). *J. Neurol. Sci.* 100:9-13.

Yan L-J, Levine RL and Sohal RS (1997). *Proc. Natl. Acad. Sci. USA* 94: 11168-11172.

Young A and Skelton DA (1994). *Int J Sports Med.* 15:149-151.

Yoshida M and Ozawa E (1990). *J. Biochem* 108:748-752.

Zerba E, Komorowski TE and Faulkner JA (1990). *Am J Physiol.* 258: C429-C435.

Immobilization, Physical Activity and Rehabilitation

[1]CARMELI ELI, [2]NETZ YAEL AND [3]REZNICK Z. AVRAHAM

[1] Sackler Faculty of Medicine, Department of Physical Therapy, Tel Aviv University, Israel
[2] The Zinman College of Physical Education, Department of Gerontology, Wingate Institute, Israel
[3] The Bruce Rappaport Faculty of Medicine, Department of Anatomy and Cell Biology, Technion- Israel Institute of Technology, Israel

Summary

The gradual decline of physical activity as we age seems to be a normal phenomenon (Cannon, 1998; Carmeli & Reznick, 1994; Metter et al., 1997). Being less active and subjected to a sedentary lifestyle exposes us to a high risk of diseases associated with early aging, functional disabilities, and social handicaps. The range of aging possibilities is seen in people's unique daily lifestyles. The way an individual experiences age varies due to culture diversity, tradition, knowledge, awareness, and interrelationships between genetics, environment and behavior. The importance of physical activity, exercise, and sports during all life stages and in particular during aging is a concept that many researchers, sociologists and educators endorse. The role of physical activity in healthy aging is well accepted in terms of biological, physical, psychological, social and emotional aspects.

Today, society, and technology offer unlimited opportunities, and choices for physical education, rehabilitation and recreation for people who are aging. Moreover, scientific evidence suggests that it is never too late to start exercising.

This chapter compiles and summarizes the research findings regarding the known benefits of physical activity and exercise on healthier aging. Just by recognizing the range, the variety and size of benefits, the potential of human movements, and the importance of being active in daily life, such as walking, it is understandable why exercise should be considered as "therapy", "medicine" and a "drug" for many diseases associated with aging.

The chapter also aims to consolidate the epidemiological features of the disease of aging and the demographic profile of aging adults in the western world. The theoretical explanations for different situations such as deconditioning, immobilization, non-weight bearing activity, inactivity, morbidity, and the sedentary lifestyle associated with being old are discussed in depth, and compared to the prevention (primary, secondary, and tertiary), and the rehabilitation benefits of exercise. The different models and theories for physical activity compliance, and the implications of habitual exercise in aging are briefly presented in this chapter, and include the social, cognitive and psychological context. Scientific studies from various health disciplines suggest that regular exercise is recommended first, to prevent premature aging, and second, to prevent premature disease by benefiting the cardio-pulmonary-vascular systems, as well as the musculoskeletal (Brooks & Faulkner, 1994; Hyatt, 1996; Thompson, 1994) immune, hormonal (Carmeli et al., 1993; Fares et al., 1996), and neurological systems (Faulkner et al., 1995; Seals et al., 1994). Hence, older adults can positively affect their mobility, endurance, power, strength, flexibility and balance with physical activity and moderate exercise.

Considering exercise as a health promotion method implies that we make it risk-free. However, health professionals that promote exercise need to provide the optimum "exercise prescription" for every individual. The answers to the questions "How much is enough?" and "How much is too much?" should be provided to the consumer, along with what exercises to do and how to do them. The known risks of exercise participation appear to be insignificant and infrequent; yet, more research is needed to clarify the dosages, the contraindications, and to clear up some concerns and apprehensions for those involved in exercise for elderly people.

The Epidemiology of Aging Diseases

Life expectancy reached a record high of 80.5 years for women and 77.8 years for men in 2000. Currently, 35 million Americans in the USA, 13% of the population, are 65 years old and older. This will rise to 70 million, or 20% of the USA, in the year 2030. As we age, we are more prone to illness, and the longer we live we are more susceptible to diseases associated with aging. A few gerontologists have suggested that the two ways of growing old are usual agers and successful agers (Meusel, 1991; Palmore, 1989). The following are physical and functional facts about aging: Aging is mainly a women's issue. There are proportionally more women 70 years old and older than men. Women over the age of 70 now represent about 70 percent of the total population of seniors. Three times more women than men live in nursing homes. The population over 85 years of age is the fastest growing in the USA. In the next 50 years, the population is expected to triple to 9 million people. When a person is 65 years old, his average life expectancy is 16.8 years. In a recent health survey, about 70 percent of the seniors polled rated their health as good, or more than good, yet 80 percent of the people ages 70 and older reported one or more chronic conditions; however, only 20 percent claimed that these conditions disrupted their daily activities. The most common health problems for seniors are osteo and rheumatoid arthritis (55%), heart disorders (65%), respiratory disorders (25%), and hypertension (23%). Chronic obstructive pulmonary disease is the fourth leading cause of death. Of accidental deaths among the elderly, 50 percent are from falls. Two of the biggest reasons for falls among older people are poor vision and medications that cause light-headedness. A decrease in muscle and bone mass (sarcopenia and osteopenia) is estimated in 40 and 35 percent, respectively (Sinaki et al., 1993; Visser et al., 2000). Over 45 percent of the cancer detected is found in people more than 65 years of age. 40 percent of elderly suffer from depression, and the risk of suicide increases with age. 10 percent of the elderly population suffers from urinary incontinence. 45 percent of non-institutionalized people ages 75 and over reported some limitation of daily activity as a result of chronic conditions. 21 percent of 65 years of age and over participate in regular activity lasting more than 15 minutes (CDC 5, 1996; ACSM, 1998).

The positive health outcomes of regular activity is well published and recommended by many studies, the World Health Organization (WHO, 1992; Butler, 2000), the Disease Control and Prevention (CDC, 1996), national and federal agencies, and well being centers (NCHS, 1994).

Evidence based studies have demonstrated that physical activity has become a survival need for the elderly, and is most likely capable of providing the control that we have been seeking in treating movement dysfunction.

The outcomes of exercise participation include a long list of biological, physiological, social, and psychological benefits for the short and long term: reduce chronic disease such as osteoporosis, COPD, increase longevity and delay mortality from all causes, prevent and control cardio-pulmonary diseases, control of obesity, cholesterol, diabetes and hypertension, improve joint mobility, flexibility, balance and muscular strength, improve life satisfaction, personal growth, self esteem, and body image, reduce the incidence of cancer and falls, increase social involvements, accelerate a rapid recovery following a bout of illness, maximize the function of the immune and hormonal systems, and improve cognitive functions, reaction time and mental health (Kirkendall & Garett, 1998; Lewis & Brown, 1994; Woollacott & Tang, 1997; O'Brien, 1998).

Sarcopenia, Immobilization and Inactivity

Movement dysfunction resulting from an acute, or chronic disease is common among elderly people. Deconditioning occurs with bed rest, joint immobilization, disuse, non-weight bearing status and inactivity. Results include muscle weakness and muscle atrophy, reduce of muscle length-tension ratio, osteoporosis, fatigability, sensorimotor decline, and hospitalization (Apple, 1990; Reznick et al., 1995). The changes in the connective tissues (skeletal muscle, tendon and ligament) are most dramatic during the first week of immobilization. Furthermore, the phenomenon of Sarcopenia adds to the general debility. Sarcopenia is defined as the loss of skeletal mass that occurs with advancing age (Evans, 1995). Sarcopenia is a generic term for the loss of muscle mass, strength and quality (composition, innervation, contractibility, capillary density, fatigability and glucose metabolism). Men and women lose the same percentage of muscle mass over time, regardless of individual body type. The greatest rate of decline in muscle mass is after age 70 (Dutta & Hadley, 1995). Although hidden, Sarcopenia results in muscle weakness, reduced activity level, increased prevalence of falls, morbidity, and loss of functional autonomy (Roubenoff & Harris, 1997). The concept of declining function with age as an irreversible phenomenon has yet to be investigated. However, Sarcopenia as a normative process or disease cannot entirely explain age reduced physical activity. Neurologic, hormonal, and immunologic, as well as, nutritional status is also thought to be associated with a decline in function and incidence of Sarcopenia. Functional decline in advancing age can be a significant limiting factor in activity. What warrants investigation is whether Sarcopenia affects all skeletal muscle, and if it can be influenced, reduced or prevented. Further work is still needed on the underlying mechanical causes of Sarcopenia. Yet, some speculative biochemical propositions were proposed as crucial: the mediating factors involved in the activation of progenitor myocells (Peterson and Houle, 1997; Partridge, 1998), age related decreases in muscle protein synthesis, the role of reactive oxygen species (Weindruch 1995), and metabolic consequences including enzyme alteration, nitrogen imbalance, and impaired glucose metabolism (Kohrt and Holloszy, 1995; Evans 1997). The changes in muscle mass should reflect an imbalance between the removal of and breakdown of old and damaged muscle protein (Nair 1995). To understand the biochemical basis for Sarcopenia, one has to compare the whole body protein synthesis, and the breakdown rates in people of different ages. However, whole body protein turnover measurements are inappropriate for determining small changes in skeletal muscle protein synthesis or breakdown because muscle contributes to less then 30% of the whole body protein turnover rate. Moreover, fractional synthesis rates of myofibrillar protein are reduced in older humans (Yarasheski et al., 1993). Hence, these findings suggest that aging is associated with the reduced capacity of muscle to synthesize new proteins. The different synthesis rate among all the individual proteins found within the muscle (e.g. ribosomes, mitochondrion, sarcoplamic reticulum, enzymes, etc.) reflects on a different synthesis capacity (Proctor et al., 1998). The synthesis of a myosin heavy chain (a protein responsible for ATP hydrolysis) is reduced in old people (Dutta and Hadley, 1995). A sharp decline (40%) in mitochondrial protein synthesis rates is reported by a few invesigators (Rooyackers et al., 1996). We are also aware of the relationship between urinary creatine excretion and muscle mass, as well as the associated decline in the basal metabolic rate because of the close association between basal metabolism and muscle mass. Foster-Burns, 1999, suggest that elderly women diagnosed with Sarcopenia can benefit from a resistance training program. The recovery effect of a training program in elderly people following immobilization was significant (Maeda et al., 1993; Pastoris et al., 2000). However, the recovery of muscles after immobilization in aged animals is impaired compared with those of young animals (Zarzhevsky et al., 2001).

Rehabilitation for the Aged

The aim of geriatric rehabilitation is the restoration of physical function to the primordial level (Hoeing et al., 1994). The health care providers must have a clear understanding of the functional capabilities and the movement needs to be achieved through the rehabilitation process. The aged individual is more prone to primary and secondary movement dysfunctions. Prior to the development of rehabilitation strategy, a comprehensive assessment will provide a clearer picture of the patient's concerns, expectations, and needs (Stuck et al., 1993). A methodological assessment will help both the patient and the therapist to establish short and long term goals. The initial evaluation will cover all the functional systems effecting movement, and include, not only the musculoskeletal, cardio-pulmonary-vascular and neurological functions, but also, mental, behavioral, and functional conditions. Findings from the evaluation would suggest the indications, and the contraindications for specific rehab intervention, along with the length, and the intensity of the rehab process and possible prognosis.

According to the National Center for Health Statistics, on average, someone has a stroke in the USA every minute. One of the easiest and most important components of stroke prevention and rehabilitation is exercise. Any physical activity burns calories, so even routine activities such as grocery shopping, planting a garden, or cleaning house can be beneficial. A woman who walks at least three hours a week can reduce her risk of heart attack and stroke by 40%, and the reduction is even greater (54%) for women who walk briskly (3.5 miles an hour).

After the acute onset of the primary disability, (i.e. hip fracture, stroke, myocardial infraction, acute renal insufficiency) elderly patients require relatively prolonged bed rest and short inactivity until they are ready for more intense rehabilitation (Von Sternberg et al., 1993). Yet, regardless of the disability, the earlier the patient moves the sooner he or she can regain strength and endurance. Hence, bed mobility, bed positioning, bed transfer and limb movements should be started as soon as possible. Early mobilization during hospitalization, and regular participation in exercise after discharge is essential. The immediate intervention is mainly to prevent pressure sores, connective-tissue contractures, blood stasis and respiratory disorders. Once such complications develop, the rehabilitation process is delayed, interrupted, and secondary conditions might worsen the medical and health status. A reconditioning exercise program can and should be tailored to meet the needs of the aged patient, which can vary from frail and dependent to healthy and independent and community dwelling (Keith et al., 1995; Kane et al., 1996).

Geriatric rehabilitation is a slow process due to the variety of psychosocial, mental and physical reasons (Hoenig et al., 1997). The therapist must be patient, an active listener, sensitive to their feelings and to non-verbal communication, and be able to provide words of empathy in order to succeed in the rehabilitation. The therapist should promote the right atmosphere, respect, and love, with fun and dignity, so as to maintain and to increase the patient's self-confidence and motivation.

Preventive Rehabilitation

Efforts to restore health and prevent primary or secondary disabilities are called therapeutic rehabilitation. Rehabilitation is defined as the restoration of form and function following illness or injury, and the restoration of an individual's capability to achieve the fullest possible life compatible with his abilities and disabilities. Preventive rehabilitation focuses on physical and psychiatric rehabilitation by a variety of means, such as early detection, therapeutic exercises (strengthening exercises, balance and gait exercises, breathing exercises), indoor and outdoor environmental assessment, and adaptations for safety, family and patient education (fall prevention, using rehab technology, adaptive techniques, splints, orthotics, walking aids), health promotion, activity precautions, and functional prediction. It is necessary to promote on-going screening, follow-up, and reassessments (Carmeli et al., 2000a).

The rehabilitation team members should have a wealth of knowledge on the history, signs, symptoms, and treatment goals of the patient. The inter and multidisciplinary approach is particularly useful for geriatric rehabilitation and could include a medical geriatric physician, a physical therapist, an occupational therapist, a dietary consultant, a nurse, a social worker, an exercise physiologist, a psychologist, and a pharmacologist.

There is two conceptual models that often applied to geriatric rehabilitation: The biomedical model based on pathophysiological outcomes and the biopsychsocial model focuses on function and well-being approach.

The Known Benefits of Exercise

Elderly people can acquire two types of benefits from regular exercises: A short and long term benefit (Fiatarone et al., 1990; Morio et al., 2000; Radak et al., 1999; Sihvoncn ct al., 1998). Physical activity rcsults not only in physiological changes, but has also been suggested to produce psychological and social effects, specifically in old age (Pate et al., 1995). The positive effect that routine exercise has on the psychosocial domain, particularly effects self concept, perceived competence, internal locus of control, self esteem, stress reduction, depression and anxiety, improved quality of sleep, improved quality of life and global well being (i.e. feeling better, sense of achievement), enhanced motivation, the formation of new friendships, the development of community spirit among other older people, and an increase in overall social support and interaction (Berger, 1996; Brassington & Hicks, 1995; Brown & Harrison, 1986; Damush & Damush, 1999; McAuley & Rudolph, 1995; Netz & Jacob, 1994; Reiter & Bendov, 1997).

The broader health and physical benefits of regular exercise include significant improvements in motor function and cognitive processing speed. Among the health benefits, exercise reduced mortality rates (Sandvik et al., 1993), extended life, lowered blood pressure (Spina et al., 1993), lowered cholesterol levels (Rantanen et al., 1994), reduced fat and body weight (Davis et al., 1998; Gardner & Poehlman, 1993), and reduced the risk of certain cancers (i.e. colon cancer) (Sturgeon et al., 1993). Among the neurophysiological benefits, exercise improved cognitive skills such as memory, intelligence and reaction time (Lupinacci et al., 1993). Of the physical benefits, exercise improved joint flexibility and range of motion, improved muscular strength, mass and endurance, slowed down the osteoporotic process (Martin & Notelvitz, 1993), improved cardiovascular function (Blumenthal et al., 1989; Puggaard et al., 1994), and improved balance and coordination (Carmeli et al., 2000b; Messier et al., 2000; Topper et al., 1993).

Physical Activity Recommendations for Elderly

During the last decade, a group of experts from CDC and ACSM reviewed the pertinent scientific evidence, and came up with a clear message for the older adult public regarding physical activity. Their results suggest that older adults should accumulate 30 minutes or more of moderate-intensity physical activity on most, preferably all, days of the week, and the experts concluded that if those "... who lead sedentary lives would adopt a more active lifestyle, there would be enormous benefit ... An active lifestyle does not require a regimented, vigorous exercises program. Instead, small changes that increase daily physical activity will enable individuals to reduce their risk of chronic diseases."

REFERENCES

American College of Sports Medicine Position Stand. (1998). Exercise and physical activity of older adults. *Medicine Science and Sports Exercise* 30:992-1008.

Appell HJ. (1990). Muscular atrophy following immobilization. *Sports Medicine 10 (1):42-58.*

Berger BG. (1996). Psychological benefits of an active lifestyle: what we know and what we need to know. *Quest* 48:330-353.

Blumenthal JA., Emery CF., Madden DJ., et al. (1989). Cardiovascular and behavioral effects of aerobic exercise training in healthy older men and women. *Journal of Gerontology: Medical Sciences* 44:147-157.

Brassington GS., Hicks RA. (1995). Aerobic exercise and self-reported sleep quality in elderly individuals. *Journal of Aging and Physical Activity* 3:120-134.

Brooks SV., Faulkner JA. (1994). Skeletal muscle weakness in old age: underlying mechanism. *Medicine Science and Sports Exercise* 26:432-439.

Brown RD., Harrison JM. (1986). The effects of a strength training program on the strength and self-concept of two female age groups. *Research Quarterly* 57:315-320.

Butler RN. (2000). Fighting frailty: prescription for healthier aging includes exercise, nutrition, safety and research. *Geriatrics* 55:20-21.

Cannon JG. (1998). Intrinsic and extrinsic factors in muscle aging. *Annuls New York Academy of Science* 854:72-77.

Carmeli E., Coleman R., Omar HL., Brown-Cross D. (2000). Do we allow elderly pedestrians sufficient time to cross the street in safety? *Journal of Aging and Physical Activity* 8:51-58.

Carmeli E., Hochberg Z., Livne E., et al. (1993). Effect of growth hormone on gastrocnemius muscle of aged rats after immobilization: biochemistry and morphology. *Journal of Applied Physiology* 75:1529- 1535.

Carmeli E., Reznick AZ. (1994). The physiology and biochemistry of skeletal muscle atrophy as a function of age. *Proceeding Society Experimental Biology and Medicine* 206:103-113.

Carmeli E., Reznick AZ., Coleman R., Carmeli V. (2000). Muscle strength and mass of lower extremities in relation to functional abilities in elderly adults. *Gerontology* 46(5):245-251.

Center for Disease Control and Prevention. (1996). *A report of the surgeon general executive summary.* Chapter 5: Physical Activity and Health. Division of Nutrition and Physical Activity, MS K-46, Atlanta GA.

Damush TM., Damush JG. (1999). The effects of strength training on strength and health-related quality of life in older adult women. *Gerontologist* 39:705-710.

Davis JW., Ross PD., Preston SD., et al. (1998). Strength, physical activity, and body mass index. *Journal of American Geriatric Society* 46:274-279.

Dutta C., Hadley EC. (1995). The significance of sarcopenia in old age. *Journal of Gerontology* 50A:1-4.

Evans WJ. (1995). What is Sarcopenia? *Journal of Gerontology* 50A:5-8.

Evans W. (1997). Functional and metabolic consequences of Sarcopenia. *Journal of Nutrition* 127:S998-S1003.

Fares FA., Gruener N., Carmeli E., Reznick AZ. (1996). Growth hormone retardation of muscle damage due to immobilization in old rats. *Annuls New York Academy of Science* 786:430-443.

Faulkner JA., Brooks SV., Zerba E. (1995). Muscle atrophy and weakness with aging: contraction-induced injury as an underlying mechanism. *Journal of Gerontology* 50A:124-129.

Fiatarone MA., Marks EC., Ryan ND., et al. (1990). High-intensity strength training in nonagenarians. *Journal of American Medical Association* 263:3029-3034.

Foster-Burns SB. (1999). Sarcopenia and decreased muscle strength in the elderly women: resistance training as a safe and effective intervention. *Journal of Women Aging* 11:75-85.

Garnder AW & Poehlman ET. (1993). Physical activity is a significant predictor of body density in women. *The American Journal of Clinical Nutrition* 57: 8-14.

Hyatt G. (1996). Strength training for the aging adults. *Activities Adaptation and Aging*, 20:27-36.

Hoeing H., Mayer-OSA., Siebens H., et al. (1994). Geriatric rehabilitation: what do physicians know about it and how should they use it? *Journal of American Geriatric Society* 42:341-347.

Hoenig H., Nusbaum N., Brummel-Smith K. (1997). Geriatric rehabilitation: state of the art. *Journal of American Geriatric Society* 45:1371-1381.

Kane RL., Chen Q., Blewett LA et al. (1996). Do rehabilitative nursing homes improve the outcomes of care? *Journal of American Geriatric Society* 44:545-554.

Keith RA., Wilson DB., & Gutierrez P. (1995). Acute and sub acute rehabilitation for stroke: a comparison. *Archive of Physical Medicine and Rehabilitation* 76:495-500.

Kirkendall DT., Garett WE. (1998). The effects of aging and training on skeletal muscle. *American Journal of Sports Medicine* 26:598-602.

Kohrt WM., Holloszy JO. (1995). Loss of skeletal muscle mass with aging: effect on glucose tolerance. *Journal of Gerontology* 50:68-72.

Lewis RD., Brown JMM. (1994). Influence of muscle activation dynamics on reaction time in elderly. *European Journal of Applied Physiology* 69:344-349.

Lupinacci NS., Rikli RE., Jones C., & Ross D. (1993). Age and physical activity effects on reaction time and digit symbol substitution performance in cognitively active adults. *Research Quarterly in Exercise and Sport* 64:144-150.

Maeda H., Kimmel DB., Raab DM., Lane NE. (1993). Musculoskeletal recovery following hindlimb immobilization in adult female rats. *Bone* 14:153-159.

Martin D & Notelvitz M. (1993). Effects of aerobic training on bone mineral density of postmenopausal women. *Journal of Bone and Mineral Research* 8:931-636.

McAuley E., Rudolph D. (1995). Physical activity, aging, and psychological well-being. *Journal of Aging and Physical Activity* 3:67-96.

Messier SP., Royer TD., Craven TE., et al. (2000). Long-term exercise and its effect on balance in older osteoarthritis adults. *Journal of American Geriatric Society* 48:131-138.

Metter EJ., Conwit R., Tobin J., Fozard JL. (1997). Age-associated loss of power and strength in the upper extremities in women and men. *Journal of Gerontology: Biological Science* 52A:B267-B276.

Meusel H. (1991). Sport activity, healthy development, successful aging. *International Journal of Physical Education* 28:10-17.

Morio B., Barra V., Ritz P et al. (2000). Benefit of endurance training in elderly people over a short period is reversible. *European Journal of Applied Physiology* 81:329-336.

Nair KS. (1995). Muscle protein turnover: methodological issues and the effect of aging. *Journal of Gerontology* 50A:107-112.

National Center for Health Statistics (NCHS). (1994). Health United States, Washington, DC: Government Printing Office.

Net Y., Jacob T. (1994). Exercise and the psychological state of institutionalized elderly: a review. *Perceptual and Motor Skills* 79:1107-1118.

Obrien S. Cousins. (1998). *Exercises, aging and health: Overcoming barriers to an active old age.* Taylor and Francis, Philadelphia, US.

Palmore EB. (1989). Exercise and longevity: A review of the epidemiologic evidence. In: R. Harris and S. Harris (Eds.), *Scientific and medical research:*

*Physical activity, aging and sport*s pp. 151-156, Albany NY: Center for the Study of Aging.

Partridge T. (1998). The fantastic voyage of muscle progenitor cells. *Nature Medicine* 4:554-555.

Pastoris O., Boschi F., Verri M., et al. (2000). The effects of aging on enzyme activities and metabolite concentrations in skeletal muscle from sedentary male and female subjects. *Experimental Gerontology* 35:95-104.

Pate RR., Pratt M., Blair SN., et al. (1995). Physical activity and public health. *Journal of American Medical Association* 273 (5): 402-407.

Proctor DN., Balagopal P & Nair KS. (1998). Age-related sarcopenia in humans is associate with reduced synthetic rates of specific muscle proteins. *Journal of Nutrition* 351S-355S.

Puggaard L., Pedersen HP., Sandager E., Klitgaard H. (1994). Physical conditioning in elderly people. *Scandinavian Journal of Medicine Science and Sports* 4:47-56.

Radak Z., Kaneko T., Tahara S., et al. (1999). The effect of exercise training on oxidative damage of lipids, proteins, and DNA in rat skeletal muscle: evidence for beneficial outcomes. *Free Radical Biology Medicine* 27:69-74.

Rantanen T., Era P., Kauppinen M., & Heikkinen E. (1994). Maximal isometric muscle strength and socio-economic status, health, and physical activity in 75-year-old persons. *Journal of Aging and Physical Activity* 2:206-220.

Reiter S., Bendov D. (1997). The self-concept and quality of life of two groups of learning disabled adults living at home and in group homes. *British Journal of Development Disability* XLII(2):97-111.

Reznick AZ., Volpin G., Ben-Ari H., Silbermann M., Stein H. (1995). Biochemical and morphological studies on rat skeletal muscles following prolonged immobilization of the knee joint by external fixation and plaster cast. *European Journal of Experimental Musculoskeletal Research* 4:69-76.

Roubenoff R., Harris TB. (1997). Failure to thrive, sarcopenia and functional decline. *Clinical Geriatric Medicine* 13:613-622.

Sandvik L., Erikssen J., Thaulow E., et al. (1993). Physical fitness as a predictor of mortality among healthy, middle-aged Norwegian men. *New England Journal of Medicine* 328:533-537.

Seals DR., Taylor JA., Ng AV., Esler MD. (1994). Exercise and aging: autonomic control of the circulation. *Medicine of Science and Sports Exercise* 26:568-576.

Sihvonen S., Rantanen T., Heikkinen E. (1998). Physical activity and survival in elderly people: a five-year follow-up study. *Journal of Aging Physical Activity* 6:133-140.

Sinaki M, Khosla S, Limburg PJ, Rogers JW, Murtaugh A. (1993). Muscle strength in osteoporotic versus normal women. *Osteoporosis* 3:8-12.

Spina RJ., Ogawa T., Miller TR., et al. (1993). Effect of exercise training on left ventricular performance in older women free of cardiopulmonary disease. *The American Journal of Cardiology* 71:99-104.

Stuck AE., Siu AL., Wiedland GD., et al. (1993). Effects of a comprehensive geriatric assessment on survival, residence and function. *Lancet* 342:1032-1036.

Sturgeon SR., Brinton LA., Berman ML., et al. (1993). Past and present physical activity and endometrial cancer risk. *British Journal of Cancer* 68:584-589.

Thompson LV. (1994). Effects of age and training on skeletal muscle physiology and performance. *Physical Therapy* 74:71-81.

Topper AK., Maki BE., & Holliday PJ. (1993). Are activity-based assessment of balance and gait in the elderly predictive of risk of falling and/or type of fall? *Journal of the American Geriatric* Society 41:479-487.

Visser M., Deeg DJ., Lips P., et al. (2000). Skeletal muscle mass and muscle strength in relation to lower extremity performance in older men and women. *Journal of American Geriatric Society* 48:381-386.

Von Sternberg T., Hepburn K., Cibuzar P., et al. (1997). Post-hospital sub acute care: an example of a manage care model. *Journal of American Geriatric Society* 45:87-91.

Weindruch R. (1995). Intervention based on the possibility that oxidative stress contributes to Sarcopenia. *Journal of Gerontology* 50:157-161.

Woollacott MH, Tang PFT. (1997). Balance control during walking in the older adult: research and its implications. *Physical Therapy* 77: 646-660.

World Health Organization. (1992). *Health of the elderly: A concern for all.*

Zarzhevsky N., Carmeli E., Focus D., et al. (2001). Recovery of muscles of old rats after hindlimb immobilization by external fixation is impaired compared with those of young rats. *Experimental Gerontology.*

Exercise and Rehabilitation from Chronic Obstructive Pulmonary Disease

SCOTT K. POWERS, R. ANDREW SHANELY AND MICHAEL CICALE

Correspondence to:

Scott K. Powers
Dept. of Exercise and Sport Sciences
Center for Exercise Science
University of Florida
Gainesville, Florida 32611
telephone: 352-392-9575 (ext. 1343)
FAX: 352-392-0316
Email: spowers@hhp.ufl.edu

Summary

Chronic obstructive pulmonary disease (COPD) is an important cause of morbidity and mortality in both industrialized and developing countries. Because of the high incidence of COPD in the world population, developing science-based rehabilitation programs for COPD has been an important clinical objective in the management of COPD patients. In this regard, rehabilitation programs for COPD patients are now well established and widely accepted as a means of enhancing management of COPD patients. Major components of successful pulmonary rehabilitation programs have included whole body muscular exercise and ventilatory muscle training. While it remains unknown if pulmonary rehabilitation improves the long-term survival of COPD patients, it is clear that pulmonary rehabilitation programs improve respiratory muscle endurance, reduce the shortness of breath associated with COPD and improve the quality of life for COPD patients.

Introduction

The incidence of pulmonary diseases is increasing in countries throughout the world. Indeed, chronic pulmonary diseases are important causes of both morbidity and mortality in most nations of the modern world (Barnes, 2000). Chronic obstructive Pulmonary disease (COPD) is the most common chronic lung disease and has been the major impetus for the development of exercise-related pulmonary rehabilitation programs (Barnes, 2000; Ries, 1997). The primary purpose of this chapter is to discuss the role of both whole body exercise and training specific to respiratory muscles in COPD rehabilitation programs. We will begin with an overview of COPD with the remaining sections of the chapter focusing upon the impact of whole body exercise and respiratory muscle training on respiratory muscle function in both healthy individuals and COPD patients.

Overview of COPD

COPD is characterized by chronic expiratory airflow limitation that is not fully reversible by treatment. This increased resistance to expiratory airflow can be caused by blockage of the airway lumen, contraction of smooth muscle in the wall of airways, and/or destruction of the parenchyma of the lung (West, 1998; Murray and Nadel, 2000). In clinical practice, the term COPD is applied to patients that have chronic bronchitis, emphysema or a mixture of the two diseases.

Chronic bronchitis is characterized by a chronic cough with excessive mucus production in the bronchial tree; this excessive mucus production results in airway blockage and therefore an increase in airway resistance. Further, chronic bronchitis may also be associated with mucous gland hyperplasia resulting in a decreased diameter of airways. In general, chronic bronchitis is diagnosed by the presence of excessive mucus in the airways and compromised pulmonary airflow that is not due to specific known diseases (e.g., bronchiectasis). More specifically, chronic bronchitis is defined by a productive cough for three months in a year for two consecutive years (Cherniack and Cherniack, 1983).

The term, emphysema, comes from the Greek word meaning "overinflation". In contrast to chronic bronchitis, emphysema is not generally associated with excessive mucus production but it is characterized by permanent enlargement of the air spaces distal to the terminal bronchioles. This results in destruction of bronchiole walls and has a negative impact on expiratory airflow. Several pathologic types of emphysema have been described and are based on on the anatomic distribution of the air space enlargement and alveolar destruction with the secondary lobule (distal to the terminal bronchiole) (Murray and Nadel, 2000).

As mentioned earlier, most patients suffering from COPD have a combination of both chronic bronchitis and emphysema. One of the most common clinical manifestations of COPD involves shortness of breath (dyspnea) upon exertion. Further, COPD patients suffering from both chronic bronchitis and emphysema often experience recurrent broncho-pulmonary infections. In severe cases of COPD, arterial hypoxemia, hypercapnia, and acidosis are also present. When chronic hypoxemia and acidosis are present, pulmonary hypertension often develops because of vasoconstriction of the precapillary arterioles. As a result of the increased pulmonary vascular resistance, the workload of the right ventricle increases and right ventricle hypertrophy results. If right ventricular hypertrophy progresses, symptoms and signs of right ventricular failure and cor pulmonale will occur.

In COPD patients exhibiting advanced emphysema, the chest is hyper-inflated and the diaphragm may be flattened. The combination of hyperinflation and increased airway resistance in COPD patients results in an elevated workload placed upon respiratory muscles. If this high workload persists for several days or weeks, respiratory muscle fatigue occurs and respiratory failure may result (Cherniack and Cherniack, 1983; Murray and Nadel, 2000).

Epidemiology of COPD

In the United States, the overall prevalence of COPD in white adults (>18 years old) is approximately 2-3 percent in nonsmokers and 12-14 percent in smokers. (Centers for Disease Control and Prevention, 1996). COPD is now the fourth leading cause of death in the United States and is the only common cause of death that is increasing (Centers for Disease Control and Prevention, 1996).

Similar to the United States, there has been an increase in the incidence and the mortality from COPD in both developing and industrialized countries. (Lopez and Murray, 1998). The World Heath Organization forecasts that by 2020, COPD will rise from its current ranking as the 12th most prevalent disease worldwide to the 5th most prevalent disease. Further, the World Heath Organization predicts that COPD will increase from the 6th to the 3rd most common cause of death worldwide. (Lopez and Murray, 1998). Potential reasons for the large rise in mortality from COPD include reduced mortality from other causes (e.g., cardiovascular diseases and infectious diseases) along with an increase in cigarette smoking and environmental pollution in developing countries (Barnes, 2000).

Pulmonary Rehabilitation-definition and Benefits

Pulmonary rehabilitation for COPD patients is now well accepted as a means to manage and improve symptoms (Ries, 1997). A formal definition of pulmonary rehabilitation has been developed by the National Institutes of Health (NIH) workshop on pulmonary rehabilitation. This group reviewed the scientific evidence supporting the role of pulmonary rehabilitation in addressing both psychological and pathophysiological problems and provided the following definition: "Pulmonary rehabilitation is a multidimensional continuum of services directed to persons with pulmonary disease and their families, usually by an interdisciplinary team of specialists, with the goal of achieving and maintaining the individual's maximum level of independence and functioning in the community" (Fishman, 1994).

Recently, a joint panel of experts from the American Association of Cardiovascular and Pulmonary Rehabilitation and the American College of Chest Physicians met to discuss guidelines for pulmonary rehabilitation and to summarize the scientific evidence to support various components or desired outcomes of pulmonary rehabilitation. The panel graded the evidence for each component (e.g., ventilatory muscle training) and desired outcome (e.g., reduced dyspnea) using a rating scale based upon the strength of the scientific evidence. Table 1 summarizes the recommendations and evidence grades contained in this document (Ries, 1997). Note the high ratings for upper and lower body exercise along with respiratory muscle training.

Table 1
Summary of recommendations and guidelines and evidence grades for pulmonary rehabilitation guidelines for COPD patients. The following rating scale was used to grade the success of various components and outcomes of pulmonary rehabilitation: A = strong scientific evidence provided by well designed and conducted studies; B = scientific evidence provided by observational studies and controlled experiments with less consistent results; and C = scientific evidence is lacking but expert opinion supports the component or outcome. Data from Ries.

Components/Outcome	Conclusions/Recommendation	Grade
Lower body exercise training	Lower body exercise training improves exercise tolerance and is recommended	A
Upper body exercise training	Strength and endurance training improves arm function and should be included in pulmonary rehabilitation	B
Ventilatory muscle training (VMT)	Evidence does not support the routine use of VMT in all patients; however, VMT may be beneficial in selected patients	B
Psychological, behavioral, and educational components and outcomes	Evidence does not support the benefits of short-term psychosocial interventions; longer-term interventions may be beneficial and export opinions supports the inclusion of this intervention	C
Dyspnea	Pulmonary rehab improves dyspnea	A
Quality of Life	Pulmonary rehab improves quality of life	B
Survival	Pulmonary rehab may improve survival	C

Exercise in Pulmonary Rehabilitation: an Overview

In general, the primary goals of pulmonary rehabilitation are accomplished by enrolling patients in programs of both education and regular exercise. A major objective of the exercise component of pulmonary rehabilitation programs is to improve respiratory and locomotor muscle endurance. In the following sections we provide an overview of respiratory muscle structure and function along with the effects of ventilatory muscle training and whole body exercise on the function of both respiratory and locomotor skeletal muscles.

Ventilatory muscle training

Respiratory muscles are skeletal muscles that act upon the chest wall to increase or decrease the thoracic volume (reviewed in Powers et al., 1997a). The principal task of respiratory muscles is to expand and compress the chest wall and, therefore, move gas in and out of the lungs to maintain blood gas and pH homeostasis. Although many muscles can act as inspiratory muscles by increasing the dimensions of the chest wall, important inspiratory muscles in humans include the diaphragm, parasternal intercostals, and the external intercostals (Powers et al., 1997). Important expiratory muscles in mammals include the abdominal muscles along with the internal intercostals (Powers et al., 1997).

Because of the potential for respiratory muscle fatigue in patients with COPD, interest in the adaptability of respiratory muscles has grown in recent years. In this section we will briefly review the effects of ventilatory muscle training on respiratory muscle endurance and discuss the impact of these changes on the COPD patient. We will begin with an overview of respiratory muscle metabolic properties.

Human respiratory muscle phenotype

In humans, only the diaphragm, parasternal intercostals, internal and external intercostals, scalenes and sternocleidomastoids have been biochemically characterized. Although skeletal muscle phenotype can be categorized in numerous ways, histochemical characterization using myofibrillar adenosine triphosphatase (ATPase) activity has been the principal technique used to investigate human respiratory muscles. Using the Brooke and Kaiser (1970) myosin ATPase-based system of fiber classification, human skeletal muscle fibers have historically been separated into 3 categories: type I; type IIa; and type IIb.

The physiological importance of muscle fiber types is due to the differences in metabolic properties and maximal shortening velocity (V_{max}) between muscle fiber types. For example, compared to types IIa and IIb, human type I fibers contain the greatest oxidative capacity and lowest V_{max} (Pette and Staron, 1990). In contrast, type IIb fibers possess the highest V_{max} but contain the lowest oxidative capacity (Pette and Staron, 1990). Finally, the oxidative capacity and V_{max} of type IIa fibers are generally between type I and type IIb fiber. While most human skeletal muscles contain a mixture of all 3 fiber types, the ratio of type I to type II fibers in a muscle is often linked with the activity pattern of the muscle (Pette and Staron, 1990). For instance, in untrained (sedentary) individuals, tonically active skeletal muscles (i.e., postural muscles) possess a larger ratio of type I to type II fibers compared to phasically active (non-postural) locomotor muscles. Therefore, it is not surprising that human respiratory muscle fibers contain a high percentage of oxidative fibers (e.g., type I and type IIa fibers) and a relatively small number of type IIb fibers. Indeed, the sum of type I and type IIa fibers in the human costal diaphragm, internal intercostals and parasternal intercostals ranges between 77 and 99% of the total fiber pool (Mizuno and Secher, 1989).

Due to the difficulty in sampling human respiratory muscles, published reports of the metabolic properties of human respiratory muscles are few. Therefore, most of the data available on human respiratory muscles are measurements from diseased patients who were physically inactive due to bed-rest (Mizuno, 1991). While some studies have examined respiratory muscles obtained from healthy individuals following accidental death, measurement of muscle enzyme activity post-mortem is often compromised because of the varied and long time periods between death and tissue removal. Therefore, it is difficult to reach firm conclusions about the bioenergetic capacity of human respiratory muscles from these studies. Nevertheless, there are many well-designed animal studies that compare the metabolic properties of rat locomotor and respiratory muscles. These investigations indicate that the activity of oxidative (i.e., Krebs cycle) enzymes in young adult and sedentary rats is 35 to 65% greater in the costal diaphragm as compared with a locomotor muscle possessing similar fiber types (i.e., plantaris) (Grinton et al., 1992; Powers et al., 1994; Powers et al., 1997b). This difference in oxidative capacity between the diaphragm and locomotor muscles of untrained animals is not surprising given that skeletal muscles are metabolically plastic and adapt quickly to regular contractile activity. For instance, a caged rat has little opportunity to exercise the plantaris muscle. In contrast, the rat diaphragm is chronically active as the resting breathing rate ranges from 80-100 breaths per minute (Crossfilt and Wissicombe, 1961).

Specific respiratory muscle training

Numerous investigators have examined the effects of specific respiratory muscle training on human respiratory muscle endurance. Based upon the approach to training, these studies can be classified in two categories: 1) voluntary isocapnic hyperpnea; and 2) inspiratory resistive loading. An overview of each of these approaches to respiratory muscle training follows.

Voluntary isocapnic hyperpnea. Voluntary isocapnic hyperpnea training is accomplished by having subjects perform voluntary hyperpnea; these subjects generally maintain high target levels of ventilation for periods up to 20-30 minutes (O'Kroy and Coast, 1993; Leith and Bradley, 1976; Morgan et al., 1987). The training sessions are typically conducted 3-5 times/week and the training effect is evaluated by measuring the maximal sustainable isocapnic ventilation that can be maintained for an established time period (e.g., 10-15 minutes). Studies investigating the effects of this ventilatory muscle training technique have demonstrated that both healthy people and patients with airway disease can improve respiratory muscle endurance with this type of ventilatory muscle training (O'Kroy and Coast, 1993; Larson et al., 1999; Leith and Bradley, 1976; Morgan et al., 1987; Belman and Gaesser, 1988; Fairbarn et al., 1991; Troosters et al., 2000).

Inspiratory resistive loading. Inspiratory resistive load training is accomplished by applying loads to inspiratory muscles 3 to 5 times per week for durations ranging from 5-15 minutes. Typically, the training effect has been evaluated in one of the following two ways. One technique quantifies the training effect as the increase in time that a fixed resistive load can be tolerated. The second technique evaluates training as the improvement in the maximal resistance that can be tolerated during a specified time period. Although reports indicate that this type of training improves respiratory muscle endurance (Aldrich and Karpel, 1985; Clanton et al., 1985), several critics have argued that these findings should be interpreted with caution (Pardy et al., 1988; Belman et al., 1986). For example, with the exception of the work of Clanton et al. (1985), all of the inspiratory resistance studies cited previously have failed to control lung volume and the breathing strategy during pre- and post-training evaluation of respiratory muscle endurance. This is an important issue because individuals tolerate a slow breathing pattern during inspiratory loading compared to a fast breathing pattern. The explanation for this observation is that slow inspirations result in lower inspiratory (mouth) pressures, reduced respiratory muscle work, a reduction in the sensation of breathing effort and a slower rate of respiratory muscle fatigue development. Indeed, Belman et al. (1986) have shown that changing from the freely chosen (i.e., normal) breathing pattern to a pattern of long, slow breaths resulted in immediate improvement of respiratory muscle endurance. Therefore, all future studies employing resistive breathing as a method of respiratory muscle training should monitor and control the lung volume and breathing pattern during the pre- and post-training evaluations (Pardy et al., 1988).

Whole body exercise training and respiratory muscles: animal studies

At present, all studies investigating the effects of whole body training on cellular changes in respiratory muscles have used animal (rodent) models. In this section, we provide an overview of these studies and discuss the effects of whole body endurance exercise on both inspiratory and expiratory muscles in rodents.

Training-induced changes in inspiratory muscles. As mentioned previously, any muscle that increases the dimensions of the chest wall is classified as an inspiratory muscle. Although numerous muscles are located between the midline of the body and head that can expand the chest, only the diaphragm, parasternal intercostals, external intercostals, scalenes and sternocleidomastoids are considered important muscles of inspiration in mammals. (De Troyer and Estenne, 1988), Of these inspiratory muscles, the muscles that have received significant experimental attention in regard to exercise training-induced adaptation are the diaphragm, parasternal intercostals and external intercostals.

The diaphragm is the most important inspiratory muscle in mammals. Functionally the mammalian diaphragm is classified as two muscles (De Troyer et al., 1981; De Troyer et al., 1982): 1) the crural (dorsal) portion that inserts into the lumbar vertebrae; and 2) the costal portion that inserts into the xyphoid process of the sternum and into the margins of the lower ribs. When investigating the functional and metabolic changes of the diaphragm to exercise training, it is important to consider the crural and costal diaphragm regions as separate muscles because these divergent areas have different ventilatory responsibilities (De Troyer et al., 1981; De Troyer et al., 1982) and different metabolic properties in rats (Powers et al., 1990; Sugiura et al., 1992). Specifically, in regard to metabolic properties, the oxidative capacity of the rat costal diaphragm is ~18% higher than that of the crural diaphragm (Powers et al., 1990; Sugiura et al., 1992). Further, myosin heavy chain (MHC) isoforms differ between the two diaphragmatic regions, with the costal diaphragm containing more type I MHC and less type IIb MHC in comparison with the crural diaphragm (Sugiura et al., 1992).

It is now clear that endurance exercise training (treadmill running) results in significant increases (+10-30%) in the oxidative capacity of the rat costal diaphragm (reviewed in Powers et al., 1997a). Interestingly, some training-induced adaptations in the diaphragm can occur rapidly (i.e., within 5 days after the initiation of training) (Vincent et al., 2000). In contrast to oxidative enzymes, endurance training appears to have little effect on diaphragm glycolytic enzymes with the exception of hexokinase. Endurance training has been shown to result in significant increases in the activity of hexokinase (+20%) within the costal diaphragm (Ianuzzo et al., 1982).

Generation of adenosine triphosphate (ATP) via oxidative phosphorylation in skeletal muscle fibers results in the formation of free radicals and hydroperoxides (reviewed in Lawler and Powers, 1998; Powers and Lennon, 1999; Powers et al., 1999). It is not surprising, therefore, that skeletal muscle possesses the antioxidant enzymes, superoxide dismutase (SOD), glutathione peroxidase (GPX) and catalase (CAT), which act to reduce cellular injury caused by free radicals and hydroperoxides (reviewed in Powers and Lennon, 1999). Several reports indicate that endurance exercise training increases total SOD and GPX activity in locomotor muscles without altering CAT activity (reviewed in Powers et al., 1999). Similiarly, Powers et al. (1994) have demonstrated that endurance exercise training results in significant increases in costal diaphragm SOD and GPX activities with no change in CAT activity.

An important practical question is, do these exercise training-induced metabolic changes in the costal diaphragm improve diaphragmatic endurance? The answer to this question is yes. Indeed, recent experiments demonstrate that both long-term (10 weeks) (Vrabas et al., 1999) and short-term (5 days) (Vincent et al., 2000) treadmill running in rats improves the endurance of the costal diaphragmatic performance during a fatigue test.

Almost all studies examining diaphragmatic adaptation to endurance training have focused on the costal diaphragm. Nonetheless, it is also clear that endurance training promotes an increase in the oxidative capacity of the crural diaphragm if the training program is of sufficient intensity and duration (Powers et al., 1994). Further, endurance training has also been shown to increase the activities of antioxidant enzymes within the crural diaphragm. Although moderate intensity exercise training does not alter crural diaphragm antioxidant enzyme activity, high intensity training results in significant increases in crural SOD activity with no change in GPX activity.

The effects of endurance training on both the parasternal and external intercostals muscles have also been investigated. These studies demonstrate that the parasternal intercostals respond to 10 weeks of endurance training by a 40% increase in oxidative capacity and SOD activity (Powers et al., 1994). No data exist concerning the effects of exercise training on parasternal myosin phenotype or glycolytic capacity.

Although the action of the external intercostals on the chest wall is dependent upon lung volume, it seems likely that the external intercostals are primarily used as inspiratory muscles in rodents (De Troyer and Estenne, 1988). In this regard, Green and Reichman (1988) investigated the effects of intense endurance training on oxidative enzyme activity in rat external intercostals muscles. The training protocol resulted in increases in mitochondrial enzyme activity (oxidative capacity) ranging from ~57 to 77% above untrained controls.

Training and expiratory muscles. Important expiratory muscles in mammals include the internal intercostals and the abdominal muscles. Green and Reichman (1988) have investigated the effects of extreme endurance training on oxidative and glycolytic enzyme activities in the internal intercostal muscles. Surprisingly, exercise training had no influence on internal intercostal oxidative enzyme activity. These findings suggest that endurance exercise training in rats does not provide a sufficient stimulus to improve the oxidative capacity of the internal intercostals.

Numerous investigators have studied the effect of endurance training on the oxidative capacity of abdominal muscles. These reports demonstrate that endurance training results in small but significant increases (i.e., 10-26% improvement) in mitochondrial enzyme activity within the rectus abdominus and external obliques (Powers et al., 1997a). By comparison, exercise training does not appear to increase the oxidative capacity of the internal obliques or transverse abdominus (Powers et al., 1997a). At present, there are no reports concerning the effects of exercise training on glycolytic capacity or myosin phenotype in expiratory muscles.

The fact that endurance training results in significant improvements in oxidative capacity in rodent rectus abdominus and external oblique muscles provides evidence that these muscles are actively recruited during treadmill running and are metabolically plastic. Similar to humans, it seems possible that these muscles serve both an expiratory function as well as trunk fixation during running in rats Powers et al., 1992; Uribe et al., 1992).

Summary of training induced changes in inspiratory and expiratory muscles. Endurance exercise is commonly used to improve the exercise capacity of respiratory and locomotor muscles in COPD patients. The increased ventilatory demands of endurance exercise rapidly leads to increases in both the oxidative and antioxidant capacity of the diaphragm, parasternal intercostals, and external intercostals as well as the rectus abdominus and the external obliques. The improved metabolic profile is not without functional benefit as the diaphragm is more resistant to fatigue following both short and long-term endurance training (see Figure 1).

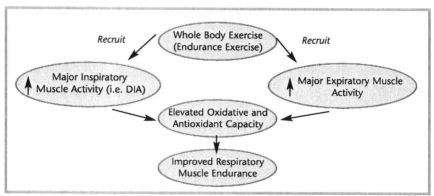

Figure 1. Overview of the effects of whole body exercise on respiratory muscle performance in animals.

Whole body exercise training and respiratory muscles: human studies

As mentioned earlier, there are no published reports regarding the effects of endurance exercise training and cellular alterations in human respiratory muscles. Instead, studies have focused upon the effects of exercise training on respiratory muscle performance. In this section, we discuss the effects of whole body exercise training on human respiratory muscle performance.

Lower body exercise. The effects of whole body exercise on human respiratory muscle strength and endurance have been investigated in both healthy individuals and individuals with obstructive airway disease. Unfortunately, analysis of these studies is often difficult because studies have used varying exercise modalities, widely different training programs and varying tests of ventilatory muscle function. However, the consensus of the literature indicates that performing lower body endurance exercise (e.g., cycling or running) results in improved ventilatory muscle endurance as evidenced by elevated maximal sustained ventilation and an increase in maximal voluntary ventilation (Troosters et al., 2000; Larson et al., 1999). Investigations comparing ventilatory performance of highly trained individuals versus untrained individuals have also concluded that whole body endurance exercise training results in an increase in respiratory muscle power output (Coast et al., 1990).

In summary, a large body of literature indicates that lower extremity training improves respiratory muscle endurance and the functional capabilities of COPD patients (reviewed in Ries, 1997). Note, however, that lower extremity training does not improve pulmonary function (reviewed in Ries, 1997).

Upper extremity training. Arm exercise training is often included in pulmonary rehabilitation programs because this type of training has the potential to improve arm exercise performance by reducing the ventilatory drive associated with upper body work and by improving the endurance of arm and shoulder muscles (reviewed in Ries, 1997). Historically, the two primary forms of arm training have been arm ergometer exercise training and progressive resistive (i.e., weight training) exercise training. Regardless of the mode of arm training, upper extremity training has been shown to improve arm function and reduce dyspnea during arm exercise in COPD patients (reviewed in Ries, 1997). Further, arm exercises appear to be safe in most COPD patients (Ries, 1997). Based upon these collective findings, strength and endurance training of the upper extremities is recommended for rehabilitation of COPD patients.

Summary and Conclusions

The importance of pulmonary rehabilitation programs for COPD patients is now well established and is widely accepted as a means of maintaining and improving function in COPD patients. Important components of successful pulmonary rehabilitation programs include whole body muscular exercise and ventilatory muscle training. Animal studies have clearly demonstrated that whole body endurance exercise training improves both respiratory muscle oxidative and antioxidant capacity. Further, human studies reveal that both whole body exercise training and ventilatory muscle training improves respiratory muscle endurance. While it is unknown if pulmonary rehabilitation increases the long-term survival of COPD patients, it is clear that whole body exercise and ventilatory muscle training programs improve respiratory muscle endurance, reduce the shortness of breath associated with COPD and elevate the quality of life for COPD patients.

Acknowledgements

This work was supported, in part, by grants from the American Lung Association-Florida, awarded to Scott K. Powers.

REFERENCES

Aldrich, T. K. and J. P. Karpel. Inspiratory muscle resistive training in respiratory failure. *American Review of Respiratory Disease* 131:461-462, 1985.

Barnes, P. J. Chronic obstructive pulmonary disease. *New England Journal of Medicine* 343:269-280, 2000.

Belman, M. J. and G. A. Gaesser. Ventilatory muscle training in the elderly. *Journal of Applied Physiology* 64:899-905, 1988.

Belman, M. J., S. G. Thomas, and M. I. Lewis. Resistive breathing training in patients with chronic obstructive pulmonary disease. *Chest* 90:662-669, 1986.

Brooke, M. H. and K. K. Kaiser. Three "myosin adenosine triphosphatase" systems: the nature of their pH lability and sulfhydryl dependence. *Journal of Histochemistry and Cytochemistry* 18:670-672, 1970.

Centers for Disease Control and Prevention. Curent estimates from the National Health Interview Survey, 1995. (DHHS publication number (PHS) 96-1527). 1996. Goverment Printing Office. Vital and Health Statistics.

Cherniack, R. M. and L. Cherniack. Respiration in health and disease. Philadelphia ; Toronto : Saunders, 1983.

Clanton, T. L., G. Dixon, J. Drake, and J. E. Gadek. Inspiratory muscle conditioning using a threshold loading device. *Chest* 87:62-66, 1985.

Coast, J. R., P. S. Clifford, T. W. Henrich, J. Stray-Gundersen, and R. L. Johnson. Maximal inspiratory pressure following maximal exercise in trained and untrained subjects. *Medicine and Science and Sports and Exercise* 22:811-815, 1990.

Crossfilt, M. and J. Widdicombe. Physical characteristics of the chest and lungs and the work of breathing in different species. *Journal of Physiology (Lond)* 158:1-14, 1961.

De Troyer, A. and M. Estenne. Functional anatomy of the respiratory muscles. *Clinics in Chest Medicine* 9:175-193, 1988.

De Troyer, A., M. Sampson, S. Sigrist, and P. T. Macklem. The diaphragm: two muscles. *Science* 213:237-238, 1981.

De Troyer, A., M. Sampson, S. Sigrist, and P. T. Macklem. Action of costal and crural parts of the diaphragm on the rib cage in dog. *Journal of Applied Physiology* 53:30-39, 1982.

Fairbarn, M. S., K. C. Coutts, R. L. Pardy, and D. C. McKenzie. Improved respiratory muscle endurance of highly trained cyclists and the effects on maximal exercise performance. *International Journal of Sports Medicine* 12: 66-70, 1991.

Fishman, A. P. Pulmonary rehabilitation research. *American Journal of Respiratory and Cricical Care Medicine* 149:825-833, 1994.

Green, H. J. and H. Reichmann. Differential response of enzyme activities in rat diaphragm and intercostal muscles to exercise training. *Journal of Neurological Science* 84:157-165, 1988.

Grinton, S., S. K. Powers, J. Lawler, D. Criswell, S. Dodd, and W. Edwards. Endurance training-induced increases in expiratory muscle oxidative capacity. *Medicine and Science and Sports and Exercise* 24:551-555, 1992.

Ianuzzo, C. D., E. G. Noble, N. Hamilton, and B. Dabrowski. Effects of streptozotocin diabetes, insulin treatment, and training on the diaphragm. *Journal of Applied Physiology* 52:1471-1475, 1982.

Larson, J. L., M. K. Covey, S. E. Wirtz, J. K. Berry, C. G. Alex, W. E. Langbein, and L. Edwards. Cycle ergometer and inspiratory muscle training in chronic obstructive pulmonary disease. *American Journal of Respiratory and Cricical Care Medicine* 160:500-507, 1999.

Lawler, J. M. and S. K. Powers. Oxidative stress, antioxidant status, and the contracting diaphragm. *Canadian Journal of Applied Physiology* 23:23-55, 1998.

Leith, D. E. and M. Bradley. Ventilatory muscle strength and endurance training. *Journal of Applied Physiology* 41:508-516, 1976.

Lopez, A. D. and C. C. Murray. The global burden of disease, 1990-2020. *Nature Medicine* 4:1241-1243, 1998.

Mizuno, M. Human respiratory muscles: fibre morphology and capillary supply. *The European Respiratory Journal* 4:587-601, 1991.

Mizuno, M. and N. H. Secher. Histochemical characteristics of human expiratory and inspiratory intercostal muscles. *Journal of Applied Physiology* 67:592-598, 1989.

Morgan, D. W., W. M. Kohrt, B. J. Bates, and J. S. Skinner. Effects of respiratory muscle endurance training on ventilatory and endurance performance of moderately trained cyclists. *International Journal of Sports Medicine* 8:88-93, 1987.

Murray, J. F. and J. A. Nadel. Textbook of respiratory medicine. Philadelphia, Saunders. 2000.

O'Kroy, J. A. and J. R. Coast. Effects of flow and resistive training on respiratory muscle endurance and strength. *Respiration* 60:279-283, 1993.

Pardy, R. L., W. D. Reid, and M. J. Belman. Respiratory muscle training. *Clinics in Chest Medicine* 9:287-296, 1988.

Pette, D. and R. S. Staron. Cellular and molecular diversities of mammalian skeletal muscle fibers. *Reviews of Physiology, Biochemistry and Pharmacology* 116:1-76, 1990.

Powers, S. K., J. Coombes, and H. Demirel. Exercise training-induced changes in respiratory muscles. *Sports Medicine* 24:120-131, 1997a.

Powers, S. K., H. A. Demirel, J. S. Coombes, L. Fletcher, C. Calliaud, I. Vrabas, and D. Prezant. Myosin phenotype and bioenergetic characteristics of rat respiratory muscles. *Medicine and Science and Sports and Exercise* 29:1573-1579, 1997b.

Powers, S. K., D. Criswell, J. Lawler, D. Martin, L. L. Ji, R. A. Herb, and G. Dudley. Regional training-induced alterations in diaphragmatic oxidative and antioxidant enzymes. *Respiration Physiology* 95:227-237, 1994.

Powers, S. K., S. Grinton, J. Lawler, D. Criswell, and S. Dodd. High intensity exercise training-induced metabolic alterations in respiratory muscles. *Respiration Physiology* 89:169-177, 1992.

Powers, S. K., L. L. Ji, and C. Leeuwenburgh. Exercise training-induced alterations in skeletal muscle antioxidant capacity: a brief review. *Medicine and Science and Sports and Exercise* 31:987-997, 1999.

Powers, S. K., J. Lawler, D. Criswell, H. Silverman, H. V. Forster, S. Grinton, and D. Harkins. Regional metabolic differences in the rat diaphragm. *Journal of Applied Physiology* 69:648-650, 1990.

Powers, S. K. and S. L. Lennon. Analysis of cellular responses to free radicals: focus on exercise and skeletal muscle. *Procedings of the Nutrition Society* 58:1025-1033, 1999.

Ries, A. L. Pulmonary rehabilitation: joint ACCP/AACVPR evidence-based guidelines. ACCP/AACVPR Pulmonary Rehabilitation Guidelines Panel. American College of Chest Physicians. American Association of Cardiovascular and Pulmonary Rehabilitation. *Chest* 112:1363-1396, 1997.

Sugiura, T., S. Morita, A. Morimoto, and N. Murakami. Regional differences in myosin heavy chain isoforms and enzyme activities of the rat diaphragm. *Journal of Applied Physiology* 73:506-509, 1992.

Troosters, T., R. Gosselink, and M. Decramer. Short- and long-term effects of outpatient rehabilitation in patients with chronic obstructive pulmonary disease: a randomized trial. *American Journal of Medicine* 109:207-212, 2000.

Uribe, J. M., C. S. Stump, C. M. Tipton, and R. F. Fregosi. Influence of exercise training on the oxidative capacity of rat abdominal muscles. *Respiration Physiology* 88:171-180, 1992.

Vincent, H. K., S. K. Powers, H. A. Demirel, J. S. Coombes, and H. Naito. Exercise training protects against contraction-induced lipid peroxidation in the diaphragm. *European Journal of Applied Physiology and Occupational Physiology* 79:268-273, 1999.

Vincent, H. K., S. K. Powers, D. J. Stewart, H. A. Demirel, R. A. Shanely, and H. Naito. Short-term exercise training improves diaphragm antioxidant capacity and endurance. *European Journal of Applied Physiology* 81:67-74, 2000.

Vrabas, I. S., S. L. Dodd, S. K. Powers, M. Hughes, J. Coombes, L. Fletcher, H. Demirel, and M. B. Reid. Endurance training reduces the rate of diaphragm fatigue in vitro. *Medicine and Science and Sports and Exercise* 31:1605-1612, 1999.

West, J. B. *Pulmonary pathophysiology: the essentials.* Baltimore, Williams & Wilkins. 1998.

Exercise-induced Bronchoconstriction in Asthma

ILDIKÓ HORVÁTH*, ÉVA HUSZÁR* AND IRÉN HERJAVECZ**

*National Korányi Institute for Pulmonology, Department of Pathophysiology, Budapest, Hungary
**VIII. Department of Pulmonology, Budapest, Hungary

Correspondence to:

Ildikó Horváth, MD, PhD
National Korányi Institute for Pulmonology
Department of Pathophysiology
Budapest PO BOX 1 Piheno u. 1
H-1529 Hungary
Phone: ++ 36 1 391-3309
Fax: ++ 36 1 394-3521
e-mail: hildiko@koranyi.hu

Summary

A common and important trigger for bronchial asthma is physical exercise. Although Exercise-Induced Bronchospasm was well-described by Sir John Floyer in the late 1600s, only during the last two or three decades have the pathophysiological and clinical characteristics of this syndrome been thoroughly examined (1). While almost all asthmatic patients develop Exercise-Induced Bronchospasm, when appropriately stressed, individuals with mild disease, especially children and adolescent, may note that this phenomenon represents the primary manifestation of their disease. In contrast, adults either with more severe asthma or with chronic obstructive lung disease may avoid the level of physical exertion that would trigger this response. The purpose of this chapter will be to describe the clinical manifestation and the pathophysiological changes that characterize Exercise-Induced Bronchospasm (EIB) in asthma, to discuss some of the proposed mechanisms responsible for this response, and to relate these findings to clinical and therapeutic considerations that are important in this syndrome.

General Considerations

The respiratory system operates over a very wide range: during peak exercise oxygen uptake rises tenfold or more, ventilation can exceed twenty times the resting minute volumes. The readjustment that occurs during and after physical exertion are of importance. The practical side of the link between exercise and the respiratory system can be readily perceived: a moderate degree of respiratory dysfunction will reduce the margin of safety without affecting the ability of the subject to live comfortably at rest or at a low level of exertion, and will only appear as the patient's inability to perform maximally within the accepted range for age and sex matched normal individuals. Many pulmonary diseases limit the capacity of the lung to adapt to increased needs for O_2 and CO_2 exchange including Chronic Obstructive Pulmonary Disease (COPD), restrictive lung conditions, Cystic Fibrosis (CF), and Asthma. In these conditions exercise capacity is limited even in moderate conditions, and the severity of the disease is partly classified by the limitation of physical exercise.

At the same time, an increasing body of knowledge points towards the beneficial effect of regular every day exercise in these conditions. Although these positive effects of regular exercise are not limited to the respiratory system, they also represent cardiac and smooth muscle adaptation; this interrelationship should be examined more in depth.

Bronchial asthma has a special connection with exercise as the limitation of lung function to parallel with the severity of asthma, and the assessment of exercise tolerance is a part of the patient's evaluation; on the other hand, there is a group of asthmatic patients presenting EIB, a phenomenon of which the underlying pathomechanism is not completely understood.

Clinical Manifestation of EIB

The bronchoconstrictor response to exercise in asthmatic subjects typically develops 5-10 min. after a short period of continuous exercise, or at a variable time after intermittent exercise; however, the latter is unlikely to cause EIB. Recovery usually occurs within 30-60 min. spontaneously (2-7). More prolonged exercise has a special place in EIB because several patients known to develop EIB claim to be able to "run through" their attack. Subsequently, there is usually a refractory period during which the response to exercise is reduced, but not that to histamine of methacholine (8, 9). The development of EIB has several similarities to the early response to allergens (for example, both are rapid in onset, and diminish in about half an hour, and are largely prevented by inhaling β2-agonists) (10). However, while the early airway responses after allergen challenge are followed by late responses in many patients, it occurs very rarely after exercise, and some investigators even deny the existence of late airway responses to exercise (11-14). Submaximal exercise insufficient to cause detectable bronchoconstriction can exert a similar refractory period like EIB (15). The bronchoconstrictor effect is influenced by the type of exercise (1,16, 17). It is greater during the night than during the day, and is aggravated by cold, damp weather, and by any condition that increases airway hyperreactivity, such as exposure to an allergen or virus infection (18-21). The effect of exercise may have a dual relationship with antigen-induced bronchospasms: bronchospasm caused by antigen exposure lead to impaired exercise performance, and on the other hand, during exercise more antigen enters into the lungs. Such changes reinforce the stimulus for bronchoconstriction although they do not necessarily increase the response (10). EIB is equally apparent in atopic and non-atopic asthmatic patients, and is viewed as part of the airway hyperreactivity in this patient group although exercise is known to produce bronchospasm in normal subjects under certain circumstances (22-25). While the airways of many patients with different lung conditions are hyperreactive to several so called "nonspecific agents", such as methacholine and histamine, hyperresponsiveness to exercise appears to be limited to asthmatic subjects, and to involve more complex pathways (26, 27).

The Mechanism of Exercise-induced Bronchoconstriction in Asthma

Physical triggers

Although the clinical manifestation of exercise-induced bronchoconstriction has been known for hundreds of years, its precise mechanism is still debated. There are several factors implicated in this airway response of asthmatic patients to exercise. The two well accepted hypotheses to explain EIB are the osmotic one and the thermal one. The first considers that inhaling large amounts of dry air during exercise leads to dehydration, and consequently, osmotic changes in the airways which initiate bronchoconstriction. The second hypothesis refers to the airway cooling during exercise, and rewarming after cessation which causes changes in microvascular blood flows resulting in airway edema causing airway narrowing. The latter hypothesis, however, was challenged by several authors who demonstrated that "mucosal dehydration" rather than heat loss is the essential pathophysiologic event for the induction of EIB. Heat and water loss eventually lead to the airway narrowing, which may be a result of muscle constriction, airway edema, and vascular congestion (28-33). These physical changes exert their effect on the airways by involving several mediators (34).

Inflammatory mediators/mechanisms

As bronchial asthma is a chronic inflammatory disease of the airways, inflammatory cells are primed and recruited into the airway. Among them mast cells, eosinophils, and basophils produce different mediators, some of which are believed to play a part in the pathomechanism of EIB (34-36).

Mast cell activation is an important step in the pathogenesis of allergen-induced acute bronchospasm, and the activation of mediator release from these cells may also participate in EIB. Mast cell activation does not necessarily require IgE-dependent pathways; in vitro, it also occurs due to osmotic challenge although this type of challenge caused only histamine release and not formation of leukotrienes (37). There are inconsistent data regarding the role of histamine in EIB. The plasma level of histamine was found to be elevated, and on the contrary to remain unchanged by EIB in asthmatic patients. This contrast, at least in part, may be explained by low levels of plasma histamine, the variability of which is influenced by many organs, and therefore, its value reflecting mast cell activation in the airways is limited (38-40). Measurements in bronchoalveolar lavage fluid represent a more direct way of sampling the airways. Bronchoscopic studies investigated the effect of hyperosmolar challenge, AMP provocation, and exercise by itself, however, failed to demonstrate exercise-induced mast cell activation in relation to EIB. The importance of histamine release in the pathomechanism of EIB was also investigated by studies using histamine (H1) receptor inhibitors. In these studies, the effect of H1-antagonists were variable and partly drug-specific (41-43). Furthermore, asthmatic subjects seemed to fit into two distinct categories based on study results: one part in which H1-antagonists provided an almost complete prevention against EIB, while in the other part, almost no prevention occurred. This observation points out that the pathological changes responsible for the development of EIB are not the same in all patients. Regarding eosinophil cells, which have a well-established role in persistent asthma, EIB was associated with an increase of Eosinophil Cationic Protein (ECP) as measured immediately after exercise, and the severity of EIB was related to baseline level of ECP in a study (44). It seems likely that eosinophils are not directly responsible for the development of EIB; they instead reflect chronic inflammatory events in asthmatic airways. Another study performed by Scollo and his coworkers demonstrated that Nitric Oxide (NO), which is known to be overproduced in the airways of asthmatic patients, is also associated with EIB, and contributes to the prolonged airway narrowing phase rather than the maximal airway narrowing evoked by exercise (45). This observation also strengthens the opinion that inflammatory mechanisms are important in the development of EIB. Furthermore, long term therapy with inhaled corticosteroids, which are known to suppress airway inflammation in asthmatic airways, also results in decreased response to exercise (46). Most likely, airway hyperreactivity and persistent airway inflammation lay down the basis for EIB, and there is a multifactorial interplay between them. Some lines of evidence point out that besides inflammatory mediators, others including adenosine, may play an important role in the development of EIB in asthma as well.

Adenosine: a broncoconstrictor mediator, which may be involved in EIB

Significantly elevated plasma concentrations of adenosine, which were found both in healthy volunteers and asthmatic patients immediately after both free-running and standardized treadmill exercises, shows that during strenuous physical exercise, overproduction of adenosine may exceed the capacity of the buffer system, which serves to eliminate the adenosine load from extracellular space (47-50). Adenosine may be released from different sources during exercise including skeletal muscles, cells developing hypoxia, and also inflammatory cells of the airways in asthmatic patients (51-54). Dehydration of the airway may be an osmotic stress on airways inflammatory cells. Eggleston *et al* demonstrated that transient osmotic stimulus resulted in the rapid release of histamine from human mast cells and basophils (55). An increase in osmosis inside the primed inflammatory cells, similar to the effect of allergen provocation (56), may also lead to the release of adenosine in asthmatic airways during exercise.

Adenosine can produce dose-related bronchoconstriction when inhaled by allergic or nonallergic asthmatics or atopic nonasthmatic subjects, but not when inhaled by healthy volunteers (57-60). It seems unlikely that *in vivo* adenosine acts directly on smooth muscle cells, rather its effect is exerted through activation of specific adenosine receptors on immunologically activated lung mast cells and circulating basophils. Activation of A3 and A2b adenosine receptors results in the release of bronchoconstrictor mediators (61-65). An exercise-induced increase in extracellular adenosine levels may result in this untoward effect, and it may be supposed that adenosine, when its level exceeds a hypothetical threshold concentration, may potentiate the effects of physical triggering factors of exercise on primed inflammatory cells, and in this way adenosine may play a role in the development of EIB (Fig 1).

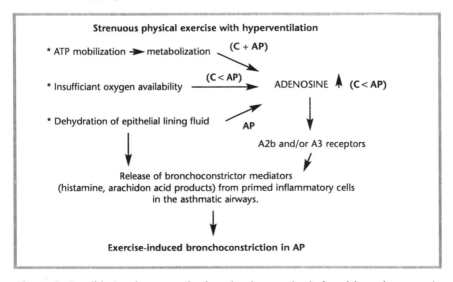

Figure 1. Possible involvement of adenosine in exercise-induced bronchospasm in asthma c: control subjects, AP: asthmatic patients.

There is now good evidence that EIB is accompanied by increases in urinary LTE4, and leukotriene receptor antagonists and lipoxygenase enzyme inhibitors have been shown to exert protective effects on EIB (66-68). On the other hand, adenosine was found to influence the allergen-induced release of histamine from isolated human mast cells, and from the actively sensitized lungs of rats (69, 70). Björck et al. observed that isolated bronchi from asthmatic patients were hyperresponsive to adenosine (71). They found that the combination of leukotriene and histamine antagonism blocked the contractile effect of adenosine, suggesting that adenosine may act on bronchial smooth muscle indirectly by facilitating histamine and leukotriene liberation. It was also shown that adenosine potentiated the antigen-induced airway obstruction, and facilitated release of histamine and bronchoconstrictor prostaglandin and thromboxane in an experimental model of asthma *in vivo* (72). Based on this observation, one might assume that in conditions when extracellular levels of adenosine are increased the effect of other factors initiating bronchospasm in asthmatic subjects may be enhanced.

Although the release of histamine and leukotrienes, and also their contribution to adenosine- and exercise-induced airway obstruction are likely different, it seems to be obvious that these two bronchoconstrictor mediators, acting directly on bronchial smooth muscle, are involved in a spasmogen effect of both challenges (73, 74). The idea of a common pathway for adenosine and exercise in developing bronchospasm in asthma has been supported by Van Schorr *et al* showing that a novel 5-lipoxygenase inhibitor could attenuate both exercise- and adenosine-induced bronchoconstriction in asthmatic patients (73). Their and others' findings indicated that leukotrienes may be involved in both exercise- and adenosine-induced airway obstruction (73, 74). There are also data showing that inhaled frusemide, which is suggested to act through increasing prostaglandin E_2 levels, can afford protection against different types of bronchoconstrictor challenges, including allergen, metabisulphite, bradykinin, and also exercise and adenosine 5' monophosphate (75, 76). Finnerty et al. found significant correlation between the change in responsiveness to adenosine 5' monophosphate (AMP) induced by repeated challenge, and the attenuation of the subsequent exercise response. They concluded that repeated challenge with AMP attenuates subsequent responsiveness to exercise, suggesting a shared mechanism of tachyphylaxis (77).

These lines of evidence implicate that adenosine may be involved in the development of EIB in asthmatic patients by acting on different cells and enhancing bronchoconstrictor mediator release. Further studies are required, however, to elucidate its precise role and the pathways involved in its effect.

Other mechanisms influenced by exercise in asthma

Very little work has been done to study the gas exchange of patients with asthma during exercise. Young et al. have examined patients with exercise-induced asthma before and after exercise using a multiple inert gas elimination technique (78). They found that despite only mild VA/Q inequality at rest, all of their subjects developed increased mismatch during the post-exercise period. At rest, VA/Q dispersion (logSDQ) increased considerably 15-28 min. after exercise, and returned to baseline 10-20 min. later. Spirometric changes followed a similar time course although these values normalized later. Arterial PO_2 reflected these changes falling to 74 mmHg, and returning to baseline later.

Thus, unlike patients with advanced stable COPD, hypoxaemia after exercise in this form of asthma is explained by worsening VA/Q inequality, and other potential factors appear secondary. This difference is not unreasonable since exercise clearly leads to increased airway obstruction in this group of asthmatic patients (78).
    Vascular mechanisms, especially changes in airway microcirculation, are also implicated in the development of EIB (79); the specific interrelationship, however, between vascular changes occurring during exercise, and the degree of airway obstruction remain unclear.

Therapeutic considerations in exercise-induced asthma (EIA)

The management of EIA begins with the assessment of asthma triggers, and other conditions the patient may have. Asthma should be distinguished from other disorders that cause respiratory symptoms during exercise, notably fixed central-airway obstruction, certain muscle disorders, exercise-induced laryngeal dysfunction, COPD and cardiac diseases.
    Not long ago, many physicians thought EIA was a variant form of the disease. Now, it is apparent that nearly all people with asthma have respiratory symptoms at least occasionally when exercising vigorously in cold, dry air. Asthmatic patients even with a mild form of the disease may have significant EIA, limiting participation in sports and recreation, and thereby impairing the quality of life. One goal of asthma therapy is to control the disease process, and maximize exercise capacity.

Exercise-induced bronchoconstriction (EIB) – the currently preferred term – as a sign of the presence of airway hyperresponsiveness to exercise suggests an overall lack of asthma control. Patients who have symptoms of asthma more than twice a week should use a medication – inhaled steroid – that offers long-term control. Although inhaled gluco-corticoids do not reduce EIB if administered as a single dose shortly before exertion, they do substantially diminish exercise-associated symptoms when administered daily as basic therapy. Therefore, long-term controller agents may have a role in treating patients with frequent symptoms of EIB.

Most drugs commonly used to treat or prevent attacks of asthma will inhibit or modify the airway responses to the physical challenge.

Inhaled β2-adrenergic agonists are the most effective medication for EIB. Preventive use of these drugs eventually protects approximately 90% of patients with EIB from the development of bronchospasm due to exercise. Traditionally, the use of a short-acting sympathomimetic agent (salbutamol, albuterol, terbutalin) 10 to 15 minutes before strenuous exertion has been the method of choice. This approach provides good prophylaxis, but the benefits only last a few hours, and repetitive dosing is required to shield against the consequences of unscheduled physical activities. With the development of sustained acting β2-agonists – salmeterol, formoterol – the duration of protection has lengthened considerably, and effective prophylaxis for 12 or more hours has become a practical reality after a single dose (80). Long acting beta-agonists are currently recommended as concomitant therapy to a controller drug for asthma, especially to prevent nocturnal awakenings. In addition, they are often used to attenuate predictable exercise-induced bronchoconstriction.

Cromolyn sodium and nedocromil sodium are also effective in preventing EIB (81). Although these drugs are known to exert their effect through mast cell stabilization, other mechanisms may also be responsible for their preventive effect of EIB. The finding that frusemide has a similar profile to sodium cromoglycate and nedocromil sodium, in terms of blocking many provocative stimuli, has improved our understanding of the possible mechanism whereby these drugs act to prevent airway narrowing. Recent studies have shown that nedocromil sodium and sodium cromoglycate block chloride ion channels in human tissue. Pharmacological agents which are capable of partly inhibiting EIB include atropine, furosemid, nifedipin, prostaglandin E_2 and heparin (82-86).

Corticosteroids, the most effective drugs in the treatment of asthma, decrease the number of inflammatory cells in the asthmatic airways, and cause an attenuation of bronchial hyperresponsiveness. The precise mechanism whereby inhaled steroids reduce the bronchial sensitivity and reactivity to physical challenges is unknown. A decrease in sensitivity may reflect an improvement in the integrity of the airway epithelium resulting in an improved mechanical barrier. Thus, nerve endings may be protected from the stimulus, and simply less mediator may reach the smooth muscle. Steroids have the potential to reduce airway oedema, and the amplifying effect that bronchial smooth muscle contraction has on airway calibre. Steroids may also improve water transport to the airway submucosa by their effect on the Na, K, and ATPase pump. By reducing the number of mast cells, steroids act to reduce the amount of bronchoconstricting mediators. In addition, by reducing the number of other inflammatory cells, the smooth muscle may become less sensitive to contractile agents in the presence of steroids (46).

Another group of agents are formed by drugs which interfere with the leukotriene pathway by inhibiting the synthesis of leukotrienes, or by antagonizing their effects through blocking the receptors (zafirlukast, zileuton, montelukast). These drugs are also effective in preventing EIB (68, 73, 74), but there is limited information to guide the practitioner on the choice of compound to use. The time to onset, the duration of action, and the relative potency of these drugs are unknown, and it is unclear whether single or repetitive dosing is required to produce an effect. Equally important, there is limited information as to whether the protection they offer is similar to that provided by more traditional forms of treatment like long acting betamimetics.

Methodological Guidelines for the Measurement of EIB

As is stated above, a wide variety of factors may influence the occurrence and the degree of EIB. Therefore, several guidelines have been set up to provide investigators with standardized method options best suited to test EIB, and to define pathomechanism, and therapeutic effects. By using these recommendations better agreement between results obtained in different laboratories can be achieved, and multicenter studies can be carried out (87-92).

Conclusions

Exercise-induced bronchoconstriction is one feature of the generalized increase in airway reactivity found in asthma. It represents an important syndrome since it may be a major disabling manifestation of the disease, or it may be an unrecognized cause of exercise-induced dyspnea. While various hypotheses exist to explain the development of bronchospasm by exercise in asthma, its precise mechanism is unknown. In spite of the controversies in the proposed mechanism underlying the development of EIB, its clinical manifestation is well-described, and the pharmacological interventions able to prevent or reduce it are usually easy and effective.

Acknowledgement

The study of the present authors on the role of adenosine in airway responses to exercise was supported by the Hungarian National Research Funding (OTKA T030340). Ildikó Horváth receives the Bolyai János Research Fellowship of the Hungarian Academy of Sciences.

REFERENCES

1. Floyer JA. (1698). *A treatise of the asthma.* London, Wilkin R and Innis W.

2. Jones RS. (1966). Assessment of respiratory function in the asthmatic child. *British Med J* 2:972-975.

3. Jones RS, Buston MH, Wharton MJ. (1962). The effect of exercise on ventilatory function in the child with asthma. *British J Diseases of the Chest* 56:78-86.

4. McNeill RS, Nairn JR, Millar JS, Ingram CG. (1966). Exercise-induced asthma. *Q J Med* 35:55-67.

5. Anderson SG, Mc Evoy JDS, Bianco S. (1972). Changes in lung volumes and airway resistance after exercise in asthmatic subjects. *Am Rev Respir Dis* 106:30-37.

6. Godfrey S. (1988). Exercise-induced asthma. In: *Allergic diseases from infancy to adulthood* (eds Bierman CW & Pearlman DS) Saunders WB, Philadelphia. 597-606.

7. Anderson SD, Silverman M, Konig P, Godfrey S. (1975). Exercise-induced asthma. *Br J Dis Chest* 69:1-39.

8. Hahn AG, Nogrady SG, Tumilty D, Laurence SR, Morton AR. (1984). Histamine reactivity during the refractory period after exercise-induced asthma. *Thorax* 39:919-923.

9. Magnussen H, Reuso G, Jones R. (1986). Airway response to methacholine during exercise induced refractoriness in asthma. *Thorax* 41:667-670.

10. Weiler-Ravel D, Godfrey S. (1981). Do exercise and antigen-induced asthma utilize the same pathways? *J Allergy Clin Immunol* 67:391-397.

11. Boulet L-P, Legris C, Turcottee H, Hebert J. (1987). Prevalence and characteristics of late asthmatic responses to exercise. *J Allergy Clin Immunol* 80:655-662.

12. Verhoeff NPLG, Speelberg B, Van Den Berg NJ, Oosthoek CHA, Stijnen T. (1990). Real and pseudo late asthmatic reactions after submaximal exercise challenge in patients with bronchial asthma. *Chest* 98:1194-1199.

13. Mc Fadden ER. (1987). Exercise and asthma. *New Engl J Med* 317: 502-504.

14. Karjalainen J. (1991). Exercise response in 404 young men with asthma: no evidence for a late asthmatic reaction. *Thorax* 46:100-104.

15. Reiff DB, Choudry NB, Pride NB, Ind PW. (1989). The effect of prolonged submaximal warming-up exercise on exercise-induced asthma. *Am Rev Respir Dis* 139:479-484.

16. Fitch KM, Morton AR. (1971). Specificity of exercise in exercise-induced asthma. *Br Med J* 4:577-581.

17. McFadden ER, Ingran RH. (1979). Exercise-induced asthma: Observations on the initiating stimulus. *N Engl J Med* 301:763-769.

18. Strauss RH, McFadden ER, Ingram RH, Deal EC, Jaeger JJ. (1978). Influence of heat and humidity on the airway obstruction induced by exercise in asthma. *J Clin Invest* 61:433-440.

19. Helenius H, Tikkanen HO, Haahtela T. (1998). Occurence of exercise-induced bronchospasm in elite runners: dependence on atopy and exposure to cold air and pollen. *Br J Sport Med* 32:125-129.

20. Arnup E, Mendella LA, Anthonisen NR. (1983). Effects of cold air hyperpnea in patients with chronic obstructive lung disease. *Am Rev Respir Dis* 128:236-239.

21. Bar-Or O, Neuman I, Dotan R. (1977). Effects of dry and humid climates on exercise-induced asthma in children and pre-adolescents. *J Allergy Clin Immunol* 60:163-168.

22. Boushey HA, Holtzman MJ, Sheller JR, Nadel JA. (1980). Bronchial hyperreactivity. *Am Rev Respir Dis* 121:389-413.

23. Bleecker ER, Chatham M, Smith PL, Rosenthal RR, Mason P, Norman PS. (1982). Airway responses to conditioned air, methacholine, histamine, and exercise in asthmatics and normals. *Am Rev Respir Dis* 125:73.

24. Paul DW, Bogard JM, Hop WC. (1993). The bronchoconstrictor effect of strenuous exercise at low temperatures in normal athletes. *Int J Sports Med.* 14:433-436.

25. Anderson SD, Holzter K. (2000). Exercise-induced asthma: Is it the right diagnosis in elite athletes? *J Allergy Clin Immunol* 106:419-428.

26. Godfrey S, Springer C, Noviski N, Maayan Ch, Avital A. (1991). Exercise but not methacholin differentiates asthma from other chronic lung diseases in children. *Thorax* 46:488-492.

27. Avital A, Springer C, Bar-Yishay E, Godfrey S. (1995). Adenosine, methacholine and exercise challenges in children with asthma or pediatric COPD. *Thorax* 50:511-516.

28. Chen WY, Horton DJ. (1977). Heat and water loss from the airways and exercise-induced asthma. *Respiration* 34:305-313.

29. Anderson SA, Daviskas E. (2000). The mechanism of exercise-induced asthma is... *J Allergy Clin Immunol* 106:453-459.

30. McNally J, Hirsch JE, Shouhrada JF. (1978). The role of hyperventilation in exercise-induced bronchoconstriction. *Am Rev Respir Dis* 118:877-884.

31. O'Byrne PM, Ryan G, Morris M, McCormack D, Jones NL, Morse JL, Hargreave FE. (1982). Asthma induced by cold air and its relation to nonspecific bronchial responsiveness to methacholine. *Am Rev Respir Dis* 125:281-285.

32. Zeballos RJ, Shturman-Ellstein R, McNally J et al. (1978). The role of hyperventilation in exercise induced bronchoconstriction. *Am Rev Respir Ds* 118:877-884.

33. O'Cain CF, Dowling NB, Slutsky AS, Hensley MJ, Strohl KP, McFadden ER, Ingram RH. (1980). Airway effects of respiratory heat loss in normal subjects. *J Appl Physiol Respir Environ Exercise Physiol* 49:875-880.

34. Larsson K, Tornling G, Gavhed D, Müller-Suur C, Palmberg L. (1998). Inhalation of cold air increases the number of inflammatory cells in the lungs of healthy subjects. *Eur Respir J* 12:825-830.

35. Lee TH, Nagakura T, Papareorgiou N, Cromwell O, Iikura Y, Kay AB. (1984). Mediators in exercise-induced asthma. *J Allergy Clin Immunol* 23:634-639.

36. Nagakura T, Lee TH, Assoufi BK, Newman-Taylor AJ, Denison DM, Kay AB. (1983). Neutrophil chemotactic factor in exercise and hyperventilation-induced asthma. *Am Rev Respir Dis* 128:294-296.

37. Eggleston PA, Kagey-Sobotka A, Proud D, Adkinson NF Jr, Lichtenstein LM (1990). Disassociation of the release of histamine and arachidonic acid metabolites from osmotically activated basophils and human lung mast cells. *Am Rev Respir Dis* 141:960-4.

38. Barnes PJ and Brown MJ. (1981). Venous plasma histamine in exercise and hyperventilation-induced asthma in man. *Clin Sci* 61:159-162.

39. Barnes PJ, Brown MJ, Silverman M et al. (1981). Circulating catecholamines in exercise and hyperventilation-induced asthma. *Thorax* 36:435-440.

40. Howarth PH, Pao GJ, Church MK, Holgate ST. (1984). Exercise and isocapnic hyperventilation-induced bronchoconstriction in asthma: relevance of circulating basophils to measurements of plasma histamine. *J Allergy Clin Immunol* 73:391-9.

41. Wiebicke W, Poynter A, Montgomery M, Chernick V, Pasterkamp H. (1984). Effect of terfenadine on the response to exercise and cold air in asthma. *Pediatr Pulmonol* 4:225-9.

42. Schachter EN, Rubin M. (1985). The effect of an aerosolized antihistamine, chlorpheniramine maleate, on exercise-induced bronchospasm. *Ann Allergy* 54:14-8.

43. Hartley JP, Nogrady SG. (1980). Effect of an inhaled antihistamine on exercise-induced asthma. *Thorax* 35:675-9.

44. Yoshikawa T., Shoji S., Fujii T., Kanazawa H., Kudoh S., Hirata K., Yoshikawa J. (1998). Severity of exercise-induced bronchoconstriction is related to airway eosinophilic inflammation in patients with asthma. *Eur Respir J* 12:879-884.

45. Scollo M, Zanconato S, Ongaro R, Zaramella C, Zacchello F, Baraldi E (2000). Exhaled nitric oxide and exercise-induced bronchoconstriction in asthmatic children. *Am J Respir Crit Care Med* 161:1047-50.

46. Waalkans HJ, van Essen-Zandvliet EEM, Gerritsen J, Duiverman EJ, Kerrebijn KF, Knol K. (1993). The effect of an inhaled corticosteroid (budenoside) on exercise-induced asthma in children. *Eur Respir J* 6:652-656.

47. Vizi É, Huszár É, Csoma Zs, Jakab Á, Böszörményi-Nagy Gy, Herjavecz I. (1998). Exercise-induced airway obstruction is related to the change of plasma adenosine concentration. *Eur Respir J* 12. (Suppl 29):47s.

48. Vizi É, Huszár É, Csoma Zs, Barát E, Böszörményi Nagy Gy, Herjavecz I, Kollai M. (2000). Role of adenosine in exercise-induced asthma. *Eur Respir J* 16 (Suppl 31):459s.

49. Schrader J, Berne RM, and Rubio R. (1972). Uptake and metabolism of adenosine by human erythrocyte ghosts. *Am J Physiol* 223(1):159-166.

50. Huszár É, Barát B, Horváth I, Kollai M. (1998). Dysfunction of adenosine buffer system in exercise-induced asthma. *Eur Respir J* 12. (Suppl 29):47s.

51. Fuller RW, Maxwell DL, Conradson T-BG, Dixon CMS, Barnes PJ. (1987). Circulatory and respiratory effects of infused adenosine in conscious man. *Br J Clin Pharmacol* 24:309-317.

52. Holgate ST, Cushley MJ, Mann JS, Hughes P, Chirch MK. (1986). The action of purines on human airways. *Arch Int Pharmacodyn* 280:240-252.

53. Mann JS, Holgate ST., Renewich AG, Cushley MJ. (1986). Airway effects of purine nucleosides and nucleotides and release with bronchial provocation in asthma. *J Appl Physiol* 61:1667-76.

54. Findley LJ, Boykin M, Fallon T, and Belardinelli L. (1986). Plasma adenosine and hypoxemia in patients with sleep apnea. *J Appl Physiol* 64(2):556-561.

55. Eggleston PA, Kagey-Sobotka A, Schleimer RP, Lichtenstein LM. (1984). Interaction between hyperosmolar and IgE-mediated histamine release from basophils and mast cells. *Am Rev Respir Dis* 130:86-9.

56. Marquardt DL, Gruber HE, Wasserman SI. (1984). Adenosine release from stimulated mast cells. *Proc Natl Acad Sci USA* 81:192-196.

57. Rafferty P, Beasley R, and Holgate ST. (1987). The contribution of histamine to immediate bronchoconstriction provoked by inhaled allergen and adenosine-5'-monophosphate in atopic asthma. *Am Rev Respir Dis* 136: 369-373.

58. Phillips GD, Rafferty P, Beasley R, and Holgate ST. (1987). Effect of oral terfenadine on the bronchoconstrictor response to inhaled histamine and adenosine-5'-monophosphate in non-atopic asthma. *Thorax* 42:939-945.

59. Phillips GD, Ng WH, Church MK, and Holgate ST. (1990). The response of plasma histamine to bronchoprovocation with methacholine, adenosine-5'-monophosphate, and allergen in atopic nonasthmatic subjects. *Am Rev Respir Dis* 141:9-13.

60. Cusley MJ, Tattersfield AE, and Holgate ST. (1983). Inhaled adenosine and guanosine on airway resistance in normal and asthmatic subjects. *Br J Clin Pharmacol* 15:161-165.

61. Polosa R, Holgate ST. (1997). Adenosine bronchoprovocation: a promising marker of allergic inflammation in asthma? *Thorax* 52:919-923.

62. Olah ME, Stiles GL. (1995). Adenosine receptor subtypes: characterization and therapeutic regulation. *Ann Rev Pharmacol Toxical* 15:581-606.

63. Ramkumar V, Stiles GL, Beaven MA, Ali H. (1993). The A3 adenosine receptor is the unique adenosine receptor which facilitates release of allergic mediators in mast cells. *J Biol Chem* 268/23:16887-90.

64. Feoktistov I, Polosa R, Holgate ST, Biaggioni I. (1998). Adenosine A2B receptors: a novel therapeutic target in asthma? *Trend Pharmacol Sci* 19(4): 148-153.

65. Forsythe P, Ennis M. (1999). Adenosine, mast cells and asthma. *Inflamm Res* 48:301-307.

66. Bronsky EA, Kemp JP, Zhang J, Guerreiro D, Reiss TF. (1997). Dose-related protection of exercise bronchoconstriction by montelukast, a cysteinyl leukotriene-receptor antagonist, at the end of a once-daily dosing interval. *Clin. Pharmacol. Ther* 62:556-561.

67. Finnerty JP, Wood-Baker R, Thomson H, Holgate ST. (1992). Role of leukotrienes in exercise-induced asthma. Inhibitory effect of ICI 204219, a potent leukotriene D4 receptor antagonist. *Am. Rev. Respir. Dis.* 145:746-749.

68. Leff JA, Busse WW, Pearlman D, Bronsky EA, Kemp J, Hendeles L, Dockhorn R, Kundu S, Zhang J, Seidenberg BC, Reiss TF. (1998). Montelukast, a leukotriene-receptor antagonist, for the treatment of mild asthma and exercise-induced bronchoconstriction. *N Engl J Med* 339:147-52.

69. Fredholm BB. (1981). Release of adenosine from rat lung by antigen and compound 48/80. *Acta Physiol Scand* 111:507-8.

70. Lee TH, Brown MJ, Nagy L, Causon R, Walport MJ, Kay AB. (1982). Exercise-induced release of histamine and neutrophil chemotactic factor in atopic asthmatics. *J Allergy Clin Immunol.* 70:73-81.

71. Björck T, Gustafsson LE, Dahlén SE. (1992). Isolated bronchi from asthmatic are hyperresponsive to adenosine, which apparently acts indirectly by liberation of leukotrienes and histamine. *Am. Rev. Respir. Dis.* 145:1087-1091.

72. Huszár É, Horváth I, Barát E, Herjavecz I, Böszörményi-Nagy Gy, Kollai M. (1998). Elevated circulating adenosine level potentiates antigen-induced immediate bronchspasm and bronchoconstrictor mediator release in sensitized guinea pigs. *J Allegy Clin Immunol* 102:687-691.

73. Van Schoor J, Joos GF, Kips JC, Drajesk JF, Carpenter PJ, Pauwels RA. (1997). The effect of ABT-761, a novel 5-lipoxygenase inhibitor, on exercise-and adenosine-induced bronchoconstricton in asthmatic subjects. *Am J Respir Crit Care Med* 155:875-880.

74. Reiss TF, Hill JB, Harman E, Zhang J, Tanaka WK, Bronsky E, Guerreiro D, Hendeles L. (1997). Increased urinary excretion of LTE4 after exercise and attenuation of exercise-induced bronchospasm by montelucast, a cysteinyl leukotriene receptor antagonist. *Thorax* 52:1030-1035.

75. Rajakulasingam K, Polosa R, Chusrch MK, Howarth PH, Holgate ST. (1994). Effect of inhaled frusemide on responses of airways to bradykinin and adenosine 5'-monophosphate in asthma. *Thorax* 49(5):485-91.

76. Pavord ID, Wisniewski A, Tattersfield AE. (1992). Inhaled frusemide and exercise induced asthma: evidence of a role for inhibitory prostanoids. *Thorax* 47:797-800.

77. Finnerty JP, Polosa R, Holgate ST. (1990). Repeated exposure of asthmatic airways to inhaled adenosine 5'-monophosohate attenuates bronchoconstriction provoked by exercise. *J Allergy Clin Immunol* 86:353-359.

78. Young IH, Corte P, Schoffel RE. (1982). Pattern and time course of ventilation-perfusion inequality in exercise-induced asthma. *Am Rev Respir Dis* 125:304-311.

79. McFadden ER. (1990). Hypothesis: exercise-induced asthma as a vascular phenomenon. *Lancet* 1:880-889.

80. Henriksen JM, Agertoft L, Pedersen S. (1992). Protective effect and duration of action of inhaled formoterol and salbutamol on exercise-induced asthma in children. *J Allergy Clin Immunol* 89:1176-1182.

81. Shaw RJ, Kay AB. (1985). Nedocromil, a mucosal and connective tissue mast cell stabilizer, inhibits exercise-induced asthma in adults. *Br J Dis Chest* 79:385-389.

82. Tinkelman DG, Cavanaugh MJ, Cooper DM. (1976). Inhibition of exercise-induced bronchospasm by atropine. *Am Rev Respir Dis* 114:87-94.

83. Ahmed T, Garrigo J, Danta I. (1993). Preventing bronchoconstriction in exercise-induced asthma with inhaled heparin. *N Engl J Med* 329:90-95.

84. Bianco C, Vaghi A, Robuschi M, Pasargiklian M. (1988). Prevention of exercise-induced bronchoconstriction by inhaled frusemide. *Lancet* 2:252-255.

85. Barnes PJ, Wilson NM, Brown MJ. (1981). A calcium-antagonist nifedipine, modifies exercise-induced asthma. *Thorax* 36:726-730.

86. Melillo E, Woolley KL, Manning PJ, Watson RM, O,Byrne PM. (1994). Effect of inhaled PGE2 on exercise-induced bronchoconstriction in asthmatic subjects. *Am J Respir Crit Care Med* 149:1138-1141.

87. Eggleston PA, Guerrant JL. (1976). A standardized method of evaluating exercise-induced asthma. *J Allergy Clin Invest* 58:414-425.

88. Eggleston PA, Rosenthal RR, Anderson SA, Anderton R, Bierman CW, Bleecker ER, Chai H, Cropp GJ, Johnson JD, Konig P, Morse J, Smith LJ, Summers RJ, Trautlein JJ. (1979). Guidelines for the methodology of exercise challenge testing of asthmatics. *J Allergy Clin Immunol* 64:642-645.

89. Haby MM, Peat JK, Mellis CM, Anderson SD, Wolcock AJ. (1995). An exercise challenge for epidemiological studies of childhood asthma: validity and repeatability. *Eur Respir J* 8:729-736.

90. Crapo RO, Casaburi R, Coates AL, Enright PL, Hankinson H, Irvin CG, MacIntyre NR, McKay RT, Wanger JS, Anderson SD, Cockcroft DW, Fish JE, Sterk PJ. (2000). Guidelines for methacholine and exercise challenge testing. *Am J Respir Crit Care Med* 161:309-329.

91. Rundell KW, Wilber RL, Szmedra L, Jetkinson DM, Mayers LB, Im J. (2000). Exercise-induced asthma screening of elite athletes: field vs. Laboratory exercise challenge. *Med Sci Sports Exerc* 32:309-316.

92. Rupp NT, Brudno S, Guill MF. (1989). The value of screening for risk of exercise-induced asthma in high school athletes. *Ann Allergy* 70:339-342.

Antioxidants, Exercise and Myocardial Ischemia-Reperfusion Injury

Li Li Ji and Steve Leichtweis

Department of Kinesiology and Nutritional Science, University of Wisconsin-Madison, WI, USA

Correspondence to:

Li Li Ji, Ph.D.
Biodynamics Laboratory
2000 Observatory Drive
Madison, WI 53706, USA
Tel: 608-262-7250, Fax: 618-262-1656
email: ji@education.wisc.edu

Summary

Reactive oxygen and nitrogen species can cause oxidative damage to a variety of cellular components and play an important role in the ethiology of myocardial ischemia-reperfusion injury. The increased level of these species results in altered physiological function and can lead to necrosis. Aged heart generates enhanced level of reactive species and is susceptible to oxidative stress. Nutritional deficiency of glutathione and other critical nutritiens can weakened endogenous antioxidant levels, whereas supplementation of antioxidant may enhance myocardial protection against ischemia-reperfusion injury. Endurance training in general improves myocardial resistance to ischemia-reperfusion injury.

Introduction

Generation of reactive oxygen species (O_2^-, H_2O_2 and $\cdot OH$) and nitrogen species (NO and peroxynitrite) is known to increase after the reperfusion of previously ischemic cardiac tissue (Simpson and Lucchesi, 1987; Downey, 1990; Matheis, Sherman et al., 1992; Wang and Zweier 1996). These reactive species can cause oxidative damage to a variety of cellular components and play an important role in the etiology of myocardial ischemia-reperfusion (I-R) injury (Brown, Terada et al., 1988; Ambrosio, Zweier et al., 1991; Park, Kenekal et al., 1992). Heart functional impairment and tissue oxidative damage seen in the postischemic heart are determined by two major factors: the level of oxidant production and the antioxidant defense capacity (Simpson and Lucchesi, 1987; Downey, 1990; Kirshenbaum and Singal, 1993). After two-decades of effort there is a vast amount of information on both basic and clinical research in this area. It is neither our intention nor within my capacity to give a general review. In the present chapter, the authors wish to focus on the effect of cellular antioxidant defense on myocardial I-R injury induced by an in situ open-chest rat heart model, as having been employed in our laboratory in the past several years. In addition, the benefits and caution of exercise training due to its direct effects on the heart or indirect effects on myocardial antioxidant systems will be discussed.

The Model of Ischemic-Reperfused Rat Heart *in Situ*

Selection of experimental models

In general there are two major methods to study myocardial I-R injury, the isolated buffer- or blood-perfused heart model (a typical procedure is the Langandorf perfused heart model) and the open-chest intact heart model. The advantage of the former *in vitro* method, either using a paced working heart or non-working heart model, is that the investigators are able to control hemodynamic (such as pre-load, after-load, coronary flow rate, etc.) and chemical (such as substrate level, pH and compositions of the perfusate) conditions to which the heart is exposed. In most cases, ischemia is imposed globally in an all-or-none fashion. This method allows us to elucidate the mechanisms of injury and/or adaptation in response to imposed insult. However, a critical limitation is this model lacks neural, hormonal and circulatory inputs that may also be modulated by I-R and other factors we are interested in, such as exercise, aging, and nutritional antioxidants. Therefore, the response of heart to I-R under physiological conditions is largely unknown. In contrast to the isolated perfused heart model, the open-chest intact heart is an *in situ* model wherein systemic and coronary circulation are kept intact. Neuroendocrinary influences on the heart are also maintained such that the heart is examined under near-physiological conditions. The limitation of this model is that the heart is subjected to so many external factors that it is difficult to study its endogenous function as affected by I-R *per se*. Another problem is that ischemia can be imposed only at the regional level with this model. Unless large animals such as dog and pig are used, areas under risk cannot be easily controlled due to the variability of individual heart anatomy and the ability to develop collateral flow. Nevertheless, since our primary purpose is to study potential physiological, nutritional and pharmacological intervention on heart I-R injury, we have employed an open-chest rat heart model in all studies reported in this chapter.

Surgical Ischemia-Reperfusion procedures

Myocardial I-R was produced by the surgical occlusion and release of the main descending branch of the left coronary artery (LCA), which perfuses the major portion of the left ventricle (Ji, fu et al., 1993; Ji, Fu et al., 1994; Leichtweis, Leeuwenburgh et al., 1996; Leichtweis, Leeuwenburgh et al., 1997; Leichtweis, Leeuwenburgh et al., 2001). Rats were anesthetized and ventilated artificially at a tidal volume of ~1.1 ml/100g body wt and at a frequency of 75-85 strokes/min. The effectiveness of ventilation was confirmed with an ABL500 blood gas analyzer. The right jugular vein of the rat was cannulated with an intravenous catheter for removal of blood samples during experiments.

A lateral thoracotomy was performed to expose the heart. The main descending vessel of the LCA was looped by a single suture ~1 mm from its origin. A 1cm segment of polyethylene tube (0.9 mm, i.d.) was slid down both ends of the 6-0 suture to compress the LCA causing a reversible occlusion of the blood flow to the left ventricle. Ischemia was maintained for a period of 30-60 min varied from study to study. Reperfusion was allowed by withdrawing the compression of the tube for 15-60 min, again varied with studies. In the sham control group, the LCA was looped with suture but not occluded for the same length of time.

Figure 1 illustrates the open-chest rat heart model.

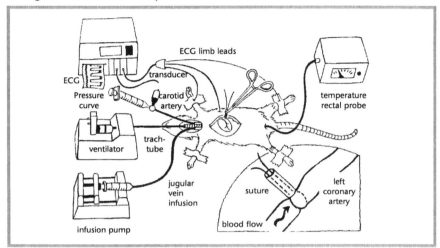

Figure 1. *Schematic illustration of the open-chest rat heart model.*

Assessment of cardiovascular function

Carotid arteries were exposed and a fluid-filled catheter (PE-50) was inserted into the right carotid artery and advanced to the left ventricular cavity. Left ventricular pressure curves were monitored using a miniature pressure transducer connected to a transducer signal conditioner. The following cardiovascular parameters were monitored in all animals throughout the entire surgery: left ventricular peak systolic (LVSP) and end-diastolic pressure (LVDP), heart rate (HR), pressure-heart rate double product (DP), left ventricular contractility ($\pm$dP/dt), and electrocardiograph (ECG).

I-R Induced Myocardial Oxidative Damage

Free radical generation

An increased free radical generation was observed in rapidly frozen ventricular tissues after I-R using the above-mentioned *in situ* intact heart model (Ji, Fu et al., 1993). Two radical signals were defined as an isotropic signal with g = 2.0038 suggestive of a semiquinone; and an anisotropic with g = 2.030 and g = 2.005 suggestive of a peroxyl radical.

Myocardial lesion

With 30-45 min ischemia in rat heart, there is likely some infarction occurring in the areas of risk (LV). Myocardial lesion was assessed by measurement of lactate dehydrogenase (LDH) release into the plasma. After ischemia LDH release was increased ~80% in LCA-occluded rats compared to sham rats. A 2.7-fold higher LDH activity was observed after reperfusion. There is a good consistency in the literature that plasma LDH (as well as creatine kinase) levels correlate well with infarction size (Simpson and Lucchesi, 1987; Downey, 1990), which is not subjected to influences by peripheral hemodynamic changes.

Lipid peroxidation

Ischemia alone had no significant effect on myocardial lipid peroxidation as measured by malondialdehyde (MDA) content, but I-R heart consistently showed higher levels of MDA compared to sham hearts (Ji, Fu et al., 1993; Ji, Fu et al, 1994; Leichtweis, Leeuwenburgh et al., 1996; Leichtweis, Leeuwenburgh et al., 1997; Coombes, Powers et al., 2000). In addition, cumene hydroperoxide levels was elevated in the I-R vs. sham hearts (Coombes, Powers et al., 2000).

Redox change

Myocardial contents of GSH and GSSG, as well as GSH/GSSG ratio, are frequently used as indicators of cellular redox status and oxidative stress in I-R hearts (Bindoli, Cavallini et al., 1988; Ceconi, Curello et al., 1988; Park, Kenekal et al., 1992). Ischemia per se did not cause a significant alteration in either GSH or GSSG content. After reperfusion LV GSH concentration was consistently found to decrease significantly below that of the sham group. I-R significantly increased myocardial GSSG content and decreased the GSH/GSSG ratio (Ji, Fu et al., 1993). It is interesting to note that I-R also decreased GSH content in RV, but had minimal effect of RV GSSG content and GSH:GSSG ratio.

Myocardial performance

HR was significantly decreased by ~18% ($P<0.01$) with the occlusion of LCA. During 30 min of ischemia, LVSP was reduced by ~75% ($P<0.01$). Initial release of LCA triggered a rapid recovery of LVSP, however, it gradually declined during reperfusion to ~80% of sham values.

Ischemia decreased +dP/dt to <25% ($P<0.01$) of pre-ischemic levels. Upon reperfusion, +dP/dt rose within 5 min to 75% ($P<0.01$) of sham values, and showed little further changes during the rest of reperfusion period. Ischemia decreased DP as a result of both decreased HR and LVSP ($P<0.01$). After 5 min reperfusion DP recovered to ~75% of sham levels ($P<0.01$). Thereafter, I-R hearts showed little improvement.

Ischemia decreased ATP concentration in LV by 50%, a decrease of ADP content and a two-fold increase in AMP conten, along with a significant reduction of myocardial energy charge (EC= ATP+1/2 ADP). Furthermore, total high-energy phosphate content was reduced by 37% (P<0.05) after I and I-R.

Ischemia caused an increase in the concentration of purine nucleotide derivatives, such as inosine monophosphate (IMP), adenosine and inosine. Adenosine rose ~8 fold above preischemic levels. No significant accumulation of nucleotide degradation products occurred after reperfusion, presumably these compounds were released into the coronary circulation (Ji, Fu et al. 1993).

GSH Deficiency and I-R Injury

The literature is divided on whether hearts depleted of endogenous GSH are more susceptible to I-R injury (Blaustein, Deneke et al., 1989; Werns, Fantone et al., 1992) or unaffected (Chatham, Seymour et al., 1988; Connaughton, Kelly et al., 1996; Verbunt, Van Dockum et al., 1996) in comparison to control hearts. However, of those studies which indicated no greater level of susceptibility to IR injury, most employed an isolated-perfused heart model which precludes an examination of plasma-tissue interaction and the inter-organ transport of GSH, potentially the most important property of GSH. The efficacy of GSH in myocardial I-R injury was investigated using an open-chest intact rat heart model. GSH levels were depleted by administration of buthionine sulfoximine (BSO). In addition, a separate group of rats received acivicin (AT125), a competitive inhibitor of γ-glutamyl transpeptidase (GGT), in addition to BSO. Hemodynamic function, myocardial and hepatic GSH status, myocardial oxidative injury and antioxidant enzymes were examined.

Hemodynamic function

HR but not DP was lower in the BSO treated rats. LVSP was constant over the 50 min in all surgical sham rats. With ischemia, LVSP decreased in all rats (P<0.01). The drop in LVSP was 39, 41 and 52%, for Saline, BSO and BSO+AT125, respectively. After I-R Saline rats regained 91% of LVSP, while BSO and BSO+AT125 rats regained 87 and 82% of their respective sham LVSP value. The difference in LVSP between sham and I-R in Saline was not significantly different, but significantly lower in BSO and BSO+AT125 **(Figure 2)**. Furthermore, LVSP after I-R was lower in BSO+AT125 than in BSO group (p<0.05). DP, product of HR and LVSP, mirrored changes observed in LVSP. Like LVSP, cardiac contractility (+dP/dt) was reduced by ischemia in all treatment groups. After reperfusion, Saline rats regained 90% of sham value (NS). However, BSO and BSO+AT125 groups regained only 76 and ~70%, respectively, of sham values (p<0.01). Thus, +dP/dt values were lower in BSO+AT125 vs. BSO or Saline (p<0.05) after I-R.

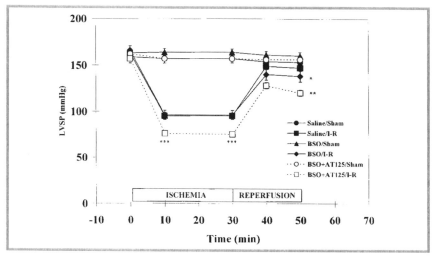

Figure 2. Response of left ventricle peak systolic pressure (LVSP) to sham and ischemia-reperfusion (I-R) in saline, buthionine sulfoximine (BSO)-treated and BSO+acivicin-treated rats. I-R, ischemia for 30 min followed by 20 min reperfusion. * P<0.05, ** P<0.01, *** P<0.001, I-R vs. Sham.

Myocardial glutathione status

As expected, BSO treatment reduced myocardial GSH content (1-2 uM). The decrease in GSH was between 48-53% (p<0.001) in both LV and RV tissue. I-R resulted in a 17-19% decrease of GSH content in the LV. A significant positive correlation was exhibited between myocardial GSH content and LVSP after 50 minutes (r=0.65, p<0.05). BSO treatment significantly reduced the GSH:GSSG ratio (p<0.05) in both LV and RV tissue. I-R significantly reduced the LV GSH:GSSG ratio (32%, p<0.01) in the Saline rats, but not in BSO or BSO+AT125 rats. In contrast to myocardial GSH, heart mitochondrial GSH levels were not affected either by BSO treatment or I-R.

Liver and kidney glutathione status

BSO treatment reduced liver GSH by 60 to 77% (p<0.01) but had no effect on GSSG levels compared to Saline rats. IR resulted in a 19 and 32% reduction (p<0.05) in liver GSH of Saline and BSO rats, but had no effect in the BSO+AT125 rats. GSSG levels was unaffected by either BSO treatment or I-R. Liver total glutathione content decreased with BSO (54%) and BSO+AT125 (70%) treatments (p<0.01). I-R resulted in a further decrease (p<0.05) in Saline and BSO but not in BSO+AT125 treated rats. BSO treatment significantly reduced GSH, GSSG and total glutathione content in the kidney (p<0.01), however, the GSH:GSSG ratio was similar between the BSO treated and Saline rats.

Antioxidant enzymes

Myocardial Cu/Zn SOD activity was elevated ($p<0.01$) in BSO+AT125 treated rats but not in Saline or BSO rats. I-R decreased Cu/Zn SOD activity (22%, $p<0.05$) in Saline but not in BSO or BSO+AT125 rats. Thus, CuZn SOD activity was higher in I-R hearts from BSO and BSO+AT125 rats than from Saline rats. Myocardial Mn SOD activity was increased ($p<0.1$) as a result of BSO treatment compared to Saline rats. However, I-R suppressed Mn SOD activity in the BSO (39%, $p<0.01$) and BSO+AT125 rats. Finally, myocardial total SOD activity increased (21%, $p<0.05$) in BSO+AT125 rats, while I-R decreased total SOD activity in Saline but not in the BSO treated rats. Myocardial activity of GSH-related enzymes GPX, GR, GST and GGT were not affected by either drug or I-R treatments.

Myocardial lipid peroxidation

Myocardial MDA content in the sham hearts was not altered by drug treatment. However, I-R significantly increased MDA levels (40%, $p<0.05$) in BSO rats but not in Saline or BSO+AT125 rats.

The most important finding of the present study was that the GSH-depleted heart displayed lower cardiac contractility, left ventricular pressure and left ventricular work as compared to GSH-adequate heart as a result of I-R. Furthermore, when cross-membrane transport of GSH was blocked by acivicin in addition to inhibition of GSH synthesis by BSO, cardiac dysfunction after 20 minutes of ischemia and 30 minutes of reperfusion was more severe than in BSO treated rats alone. These data provided strong evidence that maintenance of GSH homeostasis plays a critical role in protecting an intact heart from reperfusion injury. Further, liver GSH efflux occurred as a result of I-R potentially providing critical protection for the myocardium. Therefore, the GSH-depleted heart was at greater risk of I-R injury because systemic antioxidant support for the heart was diminished by BSO treatment.

I-R Injury and Antioxidant Supplementation

Several previous studies have attempted to look at sulfhydryl supplementation in either isolated, buffer-perfused heart models (Ceconi, Curello et al., 1988; Ferrari, Ceconi et al., 1991; Tang, Sun et al., 1991; Menasche, Grousset et al., 1992; Holdefer, Wicomb et al., 1994; Brunet, Boily et al., 1995; Chen, Gabel et al., 1995; Mass, Pirazzi et al., 1995; Seiler, Kehrer et al., 1996) or in *in vivo* heart models (Singh, Lee et al., 1989; Alberola, Such et al., 1991; Guarnieri, Turinetto et al., 1993; Kreiter, Bauer et al., 1994). These studies suggest that GSH, N-acetylcysteine (NAC), and L-2-oxothiazolidine-4-carboxylate (OTC) appear the most promising in the recovery of post-ischemic cardiovascular function and reduction of markers of oxidative and cellular damage (Ceconi, Curello et al., 1988; Singh, Lee et al., 1989; Guarnieri, Turinetto et al., 1993; Seiler, Kehrer et al., 1996). Recently, it was reported in an isolated, buffer-perfused rat heart model that GSH supplementation was able to reduce levels of peroxynitrite by forming the nitric oxide donor, S-nitrosoglutathione, following I-R injury (Cheung and Schulz 1997). Further, NAC has been shown to have direct oxidant scavenging properties in an isolated perfused heart model against hydroxyl radicals (Brunet, Boily et al., 1995) and *in vitro* hypochlorous acid (Aruomo, HZalliwell et al., 1989). However, none of the studies to date have attempted to study the overall, whole-body response to sulfhydryl supplementation and regional, myocardial I-R injury.

Infusion of sulfhydryl compounds with this in situ I-R model had to be approached with care. Pilot work indicated that infusing GSH at levels used in other studies had deleterious effects on the cardiovascular function in the current open-chest *in vivo* model, most likely the result of glutathionuria. Glutathionuria causes plasma acidosis which, in turn, can negatively impact cardiovascular and renal function (Meister, Griffith et al., 1979; Anderson and Meister, 1986). We found that a 25mM GSH stock was the highest concentration possible that did not negatively impact cardiovascular function over 75 minutes of sham surgery. Concentrations for NAC and OTC were the same to allow for adequate comparison of supplementation effects. Although many *in vitro* studies (Ceconi, Curello et al., 1988; Singh, Lee et al., 1989) have used higher concentrations of GSH, NAC, and OTC than were used in the current study, those concentrations would have been detrimental in the open-chest in vivo heart model.

GSH supplementation

Hemodynamic function

Over the course of the 75 minute procedure there was a significant linear decrease in the HR for all supplementation groups, however, LVSP and ±dP/dt remained stable in all supplemented rats subjected to the sham surgical procedure over the entire 75 minute procedure. I-R decreased HR in Saline and NAC-treated rats but not in the GSH or OTC-treated rats. Following 45 minutes of ischemia, LVSP was significantly decreased in all treatment groups. After 5 minutes after reperfusion, all groups showed an immediate increase in LVSP, regaining 86-94% of their respective sham values. However, over the course of 30 minutes of reperfusion, LVSP in the GSH-treated rats decreased significantly. Changes in the –dP/dt and DP were similar to those observed for LVSP.

Myocardial glutathione status

None of the supplementation treatments had an effect on myocardial GSH levels in the surgical shams. However, I-R significantly decreased GSH content in all treatments except the OTC-treated rats. Further, I-R reduced GSSG content in the left ventricle but not right ventricle tissue of these same groups.

Total glutathione content in left and right ventricular tissue was unchanged as a result of supplementation but I-R decreased the total glutathione levels in left ventricle tissue regardless of supplementation. Interestingly, there was a modest increase in the GSH: GSSG ratio in both the left and right ventricles as a result of supplementation, due in part to lower GSSG levels in the supplemented rats. Finally, I-R caused an unexpected increase in the GSH:GSSG ratio in the left ventricle of the OTC–treated rats, whereas GSH and NAC-treated rats showed no change, and the Saline-treated rats showed a decrease.

Antioxidant enzymes

Supplementation of GSH, NAC or OTC had no effect on the activities of Mn SOD, Cu/Zn SOD and total SOD. I-R had no effect on Mn SOD activity but did result in a significant decrease in Cu/Zn SOD activity in the Saline, GSH, and NAC -treated rats but not the OTC-treated rats. Supplementation had no effect on cytosolic GPX activity, however, I-R reduced GPX activity in the GSH- and NAC- but not in the Saline or OTC-treated rats. GR and GST activities were unaffected by supplementation but I-R reduced GR activity regardless of supplementation. Whereas, the post I-R activity of GST dropped in the GSH- and NAC-treated rats but not in the Saline or OTC-treated rats.

Myocardial lipid peroxidation

Supplementation had no effect on MDA levels in the LV tissue. However, MDA levels tended to be higher following I-R in the Saline and GSH-treated rats but not the NAC or OTC-treated rats.

There are three major findings from this study. First, sulfhydryl supplementation does not appear to benefit rats subjected to I-R injury in this model. In fact, supplemented rats in this study showed greater levels of cardiovascular dysfunction at 30 min of reperfusion than non-supplemented rats. This finding directly challenges several studies that found sulfhydryl supplementation capable of alleviating I-R related cardiovascular dysfunction (Ceconi, Curello et al., 1988; Singh, Lee et al., 1989; Tang, Sun et al., 1991; Menasche, Grousset et al., 1992; Kreiter, Bauer et al., 1994; Seiler, Kehrer et al., 1996). Some of these studies (Ceconi, Curello et al., 1988; Tang, Sun et al., 1991; Menasche, Grousset et al., 1992; Seiler, Kehrer et al., 1996), but not all (Singh, Lee et al., 1989; Kreiter, Bauer et al., 1994), used an isolated, buffer-perfused heart model which might explain part of the differences found in the current study. However, preliminary results from a clinical trial using NAC following recanalization of infarcted left ventricular tissue (ISLAND trial) indicated a beneficial effect on global and regional left ventricular ejection fraction data (Sochman, Vrbska et al., 1996). While our pilot work indicated that a slow infusion of 25mM GSH stock did not negatively impact cardiovascular function over 75 minutes of sham surgery, we cannot rule out an interaction of between the I-R and supplementation treatments for the given doses. The deterioration in cardiovascular function during reperfusion may be the result of high levels of GSH and GSH analogs in the plasma adversely affecting Na^+, K^+ channels and ATPase activity in the myocardium. Second, none of the supplemented sulfhydryl compounds caused an increase in myocardial glutathione content. In fact, OTC caused a decrease in left ventricle mitochondrial GSH levels. Therefore, acute supplementation with GSH, NAC, and OTC does not enhance myocardial antioxidant status and is likely to be the major cause of cardiovascular dysfunction seen in the current in vivo studies. However, NAC and OTC did appear to prevent an increase in myocardial lipid peroxidation following I-R injury and therefore might provide protection against I-R induced oxidative stress, but this needs to be verified using more specific markers of oxidative damage.

Vitamin E and α-lipoic acid supplementation

In addition to GSH several antioxidants have demonstrated merit in reducing myocardial I-R injury using the in vivo open-chest heart model. In a recent study by Coombes et al. (Coombes, Powers et al., 2000), the combined effects of vitamin E and α-lipoic acid were investigated in the rat heart subjected to the I-R regimen similar to that used in our laboratory. Vitamin E (α-tocopherol) is a major fat-soluble chain-breaking antioxidant located in the lipid phase of cell membrane. Vitamin E concentration in the cellular membrane is rather low, about one in several thousand molecules of phospholipid. In the heart, vitamin E content was reported to be approximately 60-70 nmol/g wet wt, similar to those in the lung and liver. α-Lipoic acid is a thio-containing antioxidant. After entering the cell it is reduced to dihydrolipoic acid (DHLA), which has been shown to be an effective antioxidant to recycle vitamin E from tocopheryl radicals. Supplementation of DHLA has been previously shown to improve cardiac performance during I-R (Haramaki, Assadnazari et al., 1995).

Dietary supplementation of vitamin E (10000 IU/kg) and α-lipoic acid (1.65 g/kg) dramatically increased myocardial vitamin E concentration (~ 5 folds). However, cardiac performance measured by peak arterial pressure and rate-pressure DP did not show any improvement in response to I-R as a result of antioxidant supplementation. Furthermore, incidence of ventricular premature beats and tachycardia caused by the I-R insult did not differ significantly between supplemented and control hearts. The only benefit resulting from antioxidant supplementation in this study was a reduced level of myocardial lipid peroxidation induced by I-R. The authors concluded that combined supplementation of vitamin E and lipoic acid do not offer greater protection to I-R induced myocardial injury.

GSH-Supplementation and Training in I-R Heart

Regular physical exercise has been shown to improve myocardial resistance to both functional and biochemical impairment induced by I-R, although there are still some controversies (Libonati, Gaughan et al., 1997; Spencer, Buttrick et al., 1997; Symons, Rendig et al., 2000). Using isolated perfused hearts, several researchers have shown that training enhances the ability of the heart to preserve LV developed pressure (Bowles, Farrar et al., 1992), high-energy phosphate content (Bowles and Starnes, 1994), and Ca^{2+} homeostasis (Palmer, Thayer et al., 1998; Palmer, Lynch et al., 1999) in response to I-R. These training effects, however, were not demonstrated uniformly and some studies showed no improvement in contractile function in endurance trained rat heart (Libonati, Gaughan et al., 1997; Symons, Rendig et al., 2000). One of the major limitations with isolated perfused heart model is the removal of circulatory and neural input, which could also be critically influenced by training (Schaible and Scheuer, 1985). The length of ischemia and reperfusion may also influence the level of oxidative stress and myocardial responses.

Although GSH play a vital role in myocardial protection against I-R (Ceconi, Curello et al., 1988; Iesnefsky, Dauber et al., 1991; Ji, Fu et al., 1994), supplementation of exogenous GSH by intraperitoneal or intravenous injection has demonstrated limited and controversial effect (Tsan, White et al., 1989). A major obstacle is that high plasma GSH concentration resulting from exogenous source can pose a strong feedback inhibition on GCS and impair operation of the γ-glutamyl cycle (Deneke and Fanurg, 1989). In contrast, oral GSH ingestion has been advocated as a more effective method to increase tissue GSH concentration and redox status (Hagen, Wierzbicka et al., 1990; Bray and Taylor, 1994). Furthermore, previous studies showed that I-R and endurance training could independently increase GGT activity in rat heart (Kihlstrom, 1990; Ondrejickova, Ziegelhoeffer et al., 1993; Leichtweis, Leeuwenburgh et al., 1997). This important adaptation may facilitate GSH breakdown and transmembrane transport, resulting in increased GSH level in the cardiomyocytes, if GSH is supplemented in diet in conjunction with training. In a recent study, the effects of dietary GSH supplementation (GSH-S), endurance training (T) and the combination of the two treatments (T/GSH-S) on myocardial functional performance and oxidative damage were examined in rat heart subjected to 45 min ischemia and 30 min reperfusion using our open-chest model, compared to untrained rats fed a control diet (U/C).

Cardiovascular response

Ischemia-caused reduction of LVSP was not affected by different treatments. However, LVSP in U/C and T/C hearts recovered to 80% of their respective sham value, whereas GSH-S and T/GSH-S hearts reached 86 and 91% of that in sham, respectively. Ischemia decreased +dP/dt to <25% of pre-ischemic levels in all groups. Upon reperfusion, +dP/dt rose to ~75% of sham values in U/C, T/C, and U/GSH-S hearts. In contrast, +dP/dt in T/GSH-S hearts recovered to 87% of sham values. Thus, +dP/dt in T/GSH-S hearts was 19, 27 & 29% (P<0.05) greater than T/C, U/GSH-S and U/C, respectively **(Figure 3)**. Similar to +dP/dt, I-R induced suppression of DP was 75% of sham in U/C and T/C hearts, whereas U/GSH-S and T/GSH-S hearts increased DP to 86 and 88% (P<0.01) of their respective sham levels. Thus, T/GSH-S hearts demonstrated a greater ability to recover LVSP, contractility and work during reperfusion after the initial 45-min ischemia, compared to any of the other treatment groups. By the end of 30-min reperfusion period, LVSP and +dP/dt in T/GSH-S hearts approached those of the sham hearts.

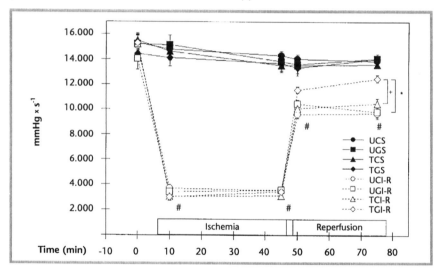

Figure 3. *Response of left ventricle contractility (+dP/dt) to ischemia-reperfusion (I-R) and sham surgery (S) in trained (T) and untrained (U) rats fed either a control (C) or GSH-supplemented diet (G). # P<0.01, I-R vs. Sham in a given time point. *P<0.05, T/G vs. U/G or U/C. + P<0.05, T/G vs. T/C.*

Cellular mechanisms underlying this increased protection observed in T/GSH-S heart may be multifaceted. Myocardial adaptations, such as enhanced high-energy phosphate reserve, high-energy phosphate content, Ca^{2+} homeostasis (Palmer, Thayer et al., 1998; Palmer, Lynch et al., 1999), coronary collateral blood flow, and antioxidant defense may play a role, but could not be entirely responsible since training alone did not elicit the benefits. Training-induced changes in GSH system were speculated to be important in that increased myocardial GGT activity along with a greater hepatic GSH output could facilitate GSH uptake by the I-R heart and thus its antioxidant capacity.

GSH Status and oxidative stress

T/GSH-S rats increased myocardial GSH content (without altering GSSG) and had a higher GSH:GSSG ratio either with sham or I-R treatment **(Figure 4)**. The net increase in GSH content was small, however, a more stable myocardial redox status might have great advantage to enzymes and proteins that are sensitive to redox disturbance. For example, Bauer et al. (Bauer, Schwarz et al., 1989) reported that pCa50 for force development was increased in skinned cardiomyocytes exposed to a higher level of GSH, whereas GSSG decreased the force by 54% at pCa 5.6. It appears that the sensitivity of contractile protein to Ca^{2+} was compromised as the intracellular environment becomes more oxidized. Turan et al. (Turan, Desilets et al., 1996) showed in rat papillary muscles that a decrease in thiol redox ratio could reduce Ca^{2+} current magnitude and hence force production. In addition, Ca^{2+} handling by intracellular organelles was hampered as shown by a rise in basal Ca^{2+} concentration and decrease in Ca^{2+} spike amplitude. The adverse effects were reversed by dithiothereitol (DTT) treatment. These mechanisms may in part explain the greater LVSP and dP/dt recovery from ischemic insult upon reperfusion in T/GSH-S heart. T/GSH-S hearts also had the lowest level of lipid peroxidation, which may benefit indirectly from a higher GSH content.

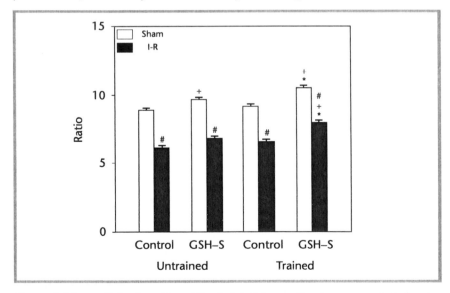

*Figure 4. Myocardial reduced to oxidized glutathione ration in response to ischemia-reperfusion (I-R) and sham in trained and untrained rats fed either a control or GSH-supplemented diet (GSH-S). # P<0.01, I-R vs. Sham . *P<0.05, trained vs. untrained. + P<0.05, GSH-S vs. Control.*

In addition to myocardial adaptations, T/GSH-S increased liver GSH content and improved plasma GSH status that facilitate myocardial protection against I-R. Higher hepatic GSH level was likely caused by increased GCS activity, the rate-limiting enzyme for GSH synthesis, with training (Meister and Anderson, 1983). This could result in a greater efflux of liver GSH, and an increase in plasma GSH concentration, presumably under the influence of vasopressin and catecholamine stimulation. Plasma GSSG levels were dramatically elevated (3-fold) by I-R, a reflection of enhanced GSSG efflux from the myocardium as well as increased ROS generated from myocardial endothelial cells (Zweier, Kuppusamy et al., 1988). T/GSH-S rats, however, demonstrated a significantly lower plasma GSSG level and higher GSH:GSSG ratio.

Myocardial necrosis

T/GSH-S increased myocardial resistance to I-R induced LDH release as a marker of necrosis. After ischemia plasma LDH activity showed 2.7 fold increase in U/C, T/C and U/GSH-S rats, compared to their sham counterparts. I-R induced LDH release was 20% lower ($P<0.05$) in T/GSH-S rats than those in other three groups. This observation suggests that fewer of the T/GSH-S hearts had suffered from myocardial infarction during I-R, and if infarction did occur, its size was probably smaller. There is a good consistency in the literature that plasma LDH (as well as creatine kinase) levels correlate well with infarction size (Simpson and Lucchesi 1987; Downey, 1990).

Antioxidant enzyme adaptation

Activities of total SOD, GPX and GR in LV were increased with training, which is consistent with previous report in rat heart with rigorous treadmill training , but not with moderate treadmill or swim training (Leewenburgh, Hollander et al., 1997; Leichtweis, Leewenburgh et al., 1997). The magnitude of induction was not affected by GSH-S. An important finding was that GGT activity in LV was elevated with T in the I-R hearts, but not sham hearts ($P<0.05$, interaction). Thus, trained hearts could have a greater potential to take up GSH from the plasma to cope with I-R induced oxidative stress, due to a higher GGT activity.

In summary, data from the present study indicate that training in conjunction with a short-term dietary GSH supplementation can enhance myocardial resistance to I-R induced damage in anesthetized rat. This important adaptation may result from a preservation of heart GSH homeostasis and increased antioxidant protection, which improved myocardial functional recovery from initial I-R insult.

I-R injury in Aged Heart

Increasing evidence suggest that aged heart generates a higher level of ROS and RNS and is susceptible to oxidative stress (Ji, 2000). Recent literature also indicates that senescent hearts may undergo some ultrastructural and biochemical changes that become more susceptible to I-R injury (Ataka, Chen et al., 1992; Lesnefsky, Gallo et al., 1994; Tani, Suganuma et al., 1997; Lucas and Szweda, 1998; Abete, Cioppa et al., 1999; Azhar, Liu et al., 1999). Whether or not postischemic injury is intensified in a senescent heart is of great scientific and clinical importance to geriatric medicine since occurrence of heart attack and stroke increase dramatically among aged population. Despite the significance of the problem, whether or not aging truly aggravates I-R damage in an intact heart under physiological condition is still uncertain. In a recent study, the interactive effects of aging and I-R on myocardial functional performance, oxidative damage and antioxidant defense was investigated using the open-chest rat heart model mentioned previously (Leichtweis et al. 2000).

Hemodynamic function in old vs. adult hearts

Aging did not seem to alter basal (preischemic) LVSP or $+dP/dt$. However, HR and DP were significantly lower in aged (24 mo) vs. young adult (6 mo) rats. Ischemia for 30 min severely suppressed hemodynamic parameters mentioned above. In general no substantial differences were seen between aged and adult hearts. After 20 min reperfusion, LVSP recovered to a great extent in aged rats heart (91% of sham) than adult (82% of sham) hearts. DP recovery was also greater in aged (90%) than adult (77%) hearts. Recovery of $+dP/dt$ after reperfusion was similar in aged and adult hearts. These data clearly demonstrate that aged hearts were not more susceptible to I-R in terms of hemodynamic function.

Our findings were in sharp contrast to several previous studies showing I-R could cause lower pressure and dP/dt recovery, greater creatine kinase release, increased myofibril damage, mitochondrial disruption and DNA fragmentation (Lesnefsky, Gallo et al., 1994, Abete, Napoli et al., 1999; Azhar, Lui et al., 1999), in aged vs. adult heart. However, lactate production was found to be similar suggesting ischemic threshold for myocardial infarction was not altered by age. The main reason for the discrepancies could be attributed to the experimental models employed. Aged hearts have shown lower high-energy phosphate reserve, less developed coronary vasculature, greater connective tissue content, and higher $Na+$ and $K+$ ion concentrations that may reduce the ischemic threshold and tolerance (Lakatta, 1993; Lesnefsky, Gallo et al., 1994). Isolated, buffer-perfused heart lacks neural and hormonal controls or blood-borne antioxidants, making them more vulnerable to I-R induced oxidative insult, whereas the in situ intact heart model used in the current study could benefit from many neural, hormonal and hemodynamic mechanisms that may be mobilized to cope with the imposed stress. For all the potential compensatory mechanisms for protection, we investigated the role of GSH antioxidant system in aged hearts.

Glutathione status

Aged hearts had higher GSH and GSSG content than adult hearts, for both LV and RV (Figure 5), but the GSH: GSSG ratio was not different. Ischemia only had little effect on GSH status regardless of age. With I-R, GSH content was decreased in both adult and aged LV, but not RV. I-R increased GSSG content in LV and RV of adult rats. In contrast, GSSG was decreased with I-R in aged hearts. I-R decreased the GSH: GSSG ratio in both LV and RV of adult rats, but had no effect on aged rats. Ischemia caused a greater increase (58% vs. 30%) in plasma GSH concentration in aged vs. adult rats, whereas plasma GSH levels were similar between the two age groups in the end of reperfusion. Higher plasma GSH levels not only provided peripheral tissues with sufficient GSH source, but could also act to scavenge superoxide and hydroxyl radicals produced in the endothelial cells of the postischemic heart (Zweier, Kuppusamy et al., 1988). In the adult rats, I-only and I-R had no effect on liver GSH. In contrast, I-R decreased liver GSH content in the aged rats, but GSSG and GSH:GSSG ratio were not altered. These data suggest that aged liver releases more GSH (26% vs. 6%) into the plasma, possibly due to augmented hormonal simulation. Aged hearts benefit from a higher plasma GSH with a greater uptake of GSH in response to I-R.

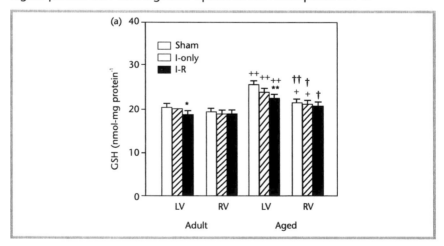

Figure 5. Myocardial glutathione (GSH) concentration in adult and aged rats during sham, ischemia (I-only), or ischemia-reperfusion (I-R) Surgery. * P<0.05, ** P<0.01, *** P<0.001, surgery effect: I-R or I-only vs. Sham. + P<0.05, ++ P<0.01, +++ P<0.001, age effect: adult vs. aged. † P<0.05, tissue effect: RV vs. LV.

Antioxidant enzymes and lipid peroxidation

Besides GSH, the aged heart appeared to have several additional advantages to alleviate oxidative stress by maintaining GSH homeostasis. First, GPX, GR and GST activities were higher in the aged heart compared to adult heart, with no decrease in SOD activity. These antioxidant enzyme adaptations may prevent ROS accumulation and excessive oxidative damage during I-R. Second, aging apparently enhanced cell's ability to export GSSG as a mechanism to maintain intracellular redox status. This was evidenced in the myocardium, where I-R resulted in a decrease rather than increase in GSSG, as shown in the adult rats. GSSG is a potentially damaging agent that promotes intra- or intermolecular protein-protein or protein-lipid cross-linkage (Meister and Anderson, 1983). Indeed, aged hearts showed similar extent of I-R induced lipid peroxidation, while GSH:GSSG ratio was kept higher compared to the adult hearts.

In summary, there are three major findings from this study. First, aged rats did not sustain any greater level of cardiovascular dysfunction in an open-chest heart model with intact circulation, compared to adult rats. Second, aged rat hearts have higher levels of GSH as well as GSH-related antioxidant enzyme activities than the adult hearts. As a result, I-R induced oxidative stress in aged hearts are not greater than that in adult hearts. Third, aged rats had a greater hepatic output of GSH into the blood, resulting in a greater plasma GSH pool for myocardial protection against oxidative stress.

Conclusion

Heart I-R injury is a complicated pathophysiological disorder due to oxidative stress caused by increased oxidant generation and insufficient antioxidant defense. Nutritional deficiency of GSH and other critical nutrients can weakened endogenous antioxidant levels, whereas supplementation of antioxidants may enhance myocardial protection against I-R. Endurance training in general improves myocardial resistance to I-R, but maximal protection can only be achieved when training is in conjunction with GSH supplementation. GSH seems to play a special role in protecting aged heart against I-R injury.

REFERENCES

Abete, P., A. Cioppa, et al. (1999). "Ischemic threshold and myocardial stunning in the aging heart." *Exp Gerontol 34* (7):875-84.

Abete, P., C. Napoli, et al. (1999). "Age-related decrease in cardiac tolerance to oxidative stress." *J Mol Cell Cardiol 31* (1):227-36.

Alberola, A., L. Such, et al. (1991). "Protective effect of N-acetylcysteine on ischaemia-induced myocardial damage in canine hearts." *Naunyn-Schmiedeberg's Archives of Pharmacology* 343:505-10.

Ambrosio, G., J. L. Zweier, et al. (1991). "The relationship between oxygen radical generation and impairment of myocardial energy metabolism following post-ischemic reperfusion." *J Mol Cell Cardiol 23* (12):1359-74.

Anderson, M. E. and A. Meister (1986). "Inhibition of gamma-glutamyl transpeptidase and induction of glutathionuria by gamma-glutamyl amino acids." *Proc Natl Acad Sci USA 83* (14):5029-32.

Aruomo, O. I., B. Halliwell, et al. (1989). "The antioxidant action of N-acetylcysteine: Its reaction with hydrogen peroxide, hydroxyl radical, superoxide, and hypochlorous acid." *Free Radical Biology and Medicine 6*: 593-7.

Ataka, K., D. Chen, et al. (1992). "Effect of aging on intracellular Ca2+, pHi, and contractility during ischemia and reperfusion." *Circulation 86* (5 Suppl): II371-6.

Azhar, G., L. Liu, et al. (1999). "Influence of age on hypoxia/reoxygenation-induced DNA fragmentation and bcl-2, bcl-xl, bax and fas in the rat heart and brain." *Mech Ageing Dev 112* (1):5-25.

Bauer, S. F., K. Schwarz, et al. (1989). "Glutathione alters calcium responsiveness of cardiac skinned fibers." *Basic Res Cardiol 84* (6):591-6.

Bindoli, A., L. Cavallini, et al. (1988). "Modification of the xanthine-converting enzyme of perfused rat heart during ischemia and oxidative stress." *Free Radic Biol Med 4* (3):163-7.

Blaustein, A., S. M. Deneke, et al. (1989). "Myocardial glutathione depletion impairs recovery after short periods of ischemia." *Circulation 80* (5):1449-57.

Bowles, D. K., R. P. Farrar, et al. (1992). "Exercise training improves cardiac function after ischemia in isolated, working rat heart." *American Journal of Physiology* 263:H804-H809.

Bowles, D. K. and J. W. Starnes (1994). "Exercise training improves metabolic response after ischemia in isolated working rat heart." *Journal of Applied Physiology 76* (4):1608-1614.

Bray, T. M. and C. G. Taylor (1994). "Enhancement of tissue glutathione for antioxidant and immune functions in malnutrition." *Biochemical Pharmacology* 47:2113-23.

Brown, J. M., L. S. Terada, et al. (1988). "Xanthine oxidase produces hydrogen peroxide which contributes to reperfusion injury of ischemic, isolated, perfused rat hearts." *J Clin Invest 81* (4):1297-301.

Brunet, J., M. Boily, et al. (1995). "Effects of N-acetylcysteine in the rat heart reperfused after low-flow ischemia: Evidence for a direct scavenging of hydroxyl radicals and a nitric oxide-dependent increase in coronary flow." *Free Radicals in Biology and Medicine 19* (5):627-38.

Ceconi, C., S. Curello, et al. (1988). "The role of glutathione status in the protection against ischaemic and reperfusion damage: effects of N-acetylcysteine." *Journal of Molecular and Cellular Cardiology* 20:5-13.

Chatham, J. C., A. L. Seymour, et al. (1988). "Depletion of myocardial glutathione: its effects on heart function and metabolism during ischaemia and reperfusion." *Cardiovasc Res 22* (11):833-9.

Chen, W., S. Gabel, et al. (1995). "A redox-based mechanism for cardioprotection induced by ischemic preconditioning in perfused heart." *Circulation Research 77* (2):424-9.

Cheung, P. Y. and R. Schulz (1997). "Glutathione inhibits peroxynitrite release and reduces myocardial ischemia-reperfusion injury." *4th Annual Meeting of the Oxygen Society Abstracts: 77.*

Connaughton, M., F. J. Kelly, et al. (1996). "Ventricular arrhythmias induced by ischaemia-reperfusion are unaffected by myocardial glutathione depletion." *J Mol Cell Cardiol 28* (4):679-88.

Coombes, J. S., S. K. Powers, et al. (2000). "Effect of combined supplementation with vitamin E and alpha-lipoic acid on myocardial performance during in vivo ischaemia-reperfusion." *Acta Physiol Scand 169* (4):261-9.

Coombes, J. S., S. K. Powers, et al. (2000). "Improved cardiac performance after ischemia in aged rats supplemented with vitamin E and alpha-lipoic acid." *Am J Physiol Regul Integr Comp Physiol 279* (6):R2149-55.

Deneke, S. M. and B. L. Fanburg (1989). "Regulation of cellular glutathione." *Am J Physiol 257* (4 Pt 1):L163-73.

Downey, J. M. (1990). Free radicals and their involvement during long-term myocardial ischemia and reperfusion. *Annual Review of Physiology.* 52:487-504.

Ferrari, R., C. Ceconi, et al. (1991). "Oxygen free radicals and myocardial damage: protective role of thiol- containing agents." *Am J Med 91* (3C): 95S-105S.

Guarnieri, C., B. Turinetto, et al. (1993). "Effect of glutathione monoethyl ester on glutathione level and cardiac energetics in reperfused pig heart." *Res Commun Chem Pathol Pharmacol 81* (1):33-44.

Hagen, T. M., G. T. Wierzbicka, et al. (1990). "Bioavailability of dietary glutathione: effect on plasma concentration." *American Journal of Physiology* 259:G524-529.

Haramaki, N., H. Assadnazari, et al. (1995). "The influence of vitamin E and dihydrolipoic acid on cardiac energy and glutathione status under hypoxia-reoxygenation." *Biochem Mol Biol Int* 37(3):591-7.

Holdefer, M. M., W. N. Wicomb, et al. (1994). "Cardiotonic effects of reduced sulfhydryl amines after preservation of rabbit hearts." *Journal of Heart and Lung Transplant* 13:157-9.

Ji, L. L., R. G. Fu, et al. (1994). "Cardiac hypertrophy alters myocardial response to ischaemia and reperfusion in vivo." *Acta Physiol Scand* 151(3):279-90.

Ji, L. L., R. G. Fu, et al. (1993). "Myocardial response to regional ischemia and reperfusion in vivo in rat heart." *Can J Physiol Pharmacol 71* (10-11):811-7.

Kihlstrom, M. (1990). "Protection effect of endurance training against reoxygenation-induced injuries in rat heart." *Journal of Applied Physiology 68* (4):1672-1678.

Kirshenbaum, L. A. and P. K. Singal (1993). "Increase in endogenous antioxidant enzymes protects hearts against reperfusion injury." *Am J Physiol 265* (2 Pt 2):H484-93.

Kreiter, H., S. F. Bauer, et al. (1994). "Infusion of oxidized glutathione enhances postischemic segment-shortening in dog hearts." *Cardioscience 5* (2):115-26.

Lakatta, E. G. (1993). "Cardiovascular regulatory mechanisms in advanced age." *Physiological Reviews 73* (2):413-67.

Leeuwenburgh, C., J. Hollander, et al. (1997). "Adaptations of glutathione antioxidant system to endurance training are tissue and muscle fiber specific." *Am J Physiol 272* (1 Pt 2):R363-9.

Leichtweis, S. and L. L. Ji (2001). "Glutathione deficiency intensifies ischaemia-reperfusion induced cardiac dysfunction and oxidative stress." *Acta Physiol Scand 172* (1):1-10.

Leichtweis, S., C. Leeuwenburgh, et al. (2001). "Aged rat hearts are not more susceptible to ischemia-reperfusion injury in vivo: role of glutathione." *Mech Ageing Dev 122* (6):503-18.

Leichtweis, S. B., C. Leeuwenburgh, et al. (1996). "Ischaemia-reperfusion induced alterations of mitochondrial function in hypertrophied rat heart." *Acta Physiol Scand 156* (1):51-60.

Leichtweis, S. B., C. Leeuwenburgh, et al. (1997). "Rigorous swim training impairs mitochondrial function in post-ischaemic rat heart." *Acta Physiol Scand 160* (2):139-48.

Lesnefsky, E. J., I. M. Dauber, et al. (1991). "Myocardial sulfhydryl pool alterations occur during reperfusion after brief and prolonged myocardial ischemia in vivo." *Circ Res 68*:605-13.

Lesnefsky, E. J., D. S. Gallo, et al. (1994). "Aging increases ischemia-reperfusion injury in the isolated, buffer- perfused heart." *J Lab Clin Med 124* (6):843-51.

Libonati, J. R., J. P. Gaughan, et al. (1997). "Reduced ischemia and reperfusion injury following exercise training." *Med Sci Sports Exerc 29* (4):509-16.

Lucas, D. T. and L. I. Szweda (1998). "Cardiac reperfusion injury: aging, lipid peroxidation, and mitochondrial dysfunction." *Proc Natl Acad Sci USA 95* (2): 510-4.

Mass, H., B. Pirazzi, et al. (1995). "N-acetylcysteine diminishes injury induced by ballon angioplasty of the carotid artery in rabbits." *Biochemical and Biophysical Research Communications 215* (2):613-8.

Matheis, G., M. P. Sherman, et al. (1992). "Role of L-arginine-nitric oxide pathway in myocardial reoxygenation injury." *Am J Physiol 262*:H616-20.

Meister, A. (1991). "Glutathione deficiency produced by inhibition of its synthesis, and its reversal; applications in research and therapy." *Pharmacol Ther 51* (2):155-94.

Meister, A. and M. E. Anderson (1983). "Glutathione." *Annual Review of Biochemistry 52*:711-760.

Meister, A., O. W. Griffith, et al. (1979). "New aspects of glutathione metabolism and translocation in mammals." *Ciba Found Symp* (72):135-61.

Menasche, P., C. Grousset, et al. (1992). "Maintenance of the myocardial thiol pool by N-acetylcysteine. An effective means of improving cardioplegic protection." *J Thorac Cardiovasc Surg 103* (5):936-44.

Ondrejickova, O., A. Ziegelhoeffer, et al. (1993). "Evaluation of ischemia-reperfusion injury by malondialdehyde, glutathione and gamma-glutamyl transpeptidase: lack of specific local effects in diverse parts of the dog heart following acute coronary occlusion." *Cardioscience 4* (4):225-30.

Palmer, B. M., J. M. Lynch, et al. (1999). "Effects of chronic run training on Na+-dependent Ca2+ efflux from rat left ventricular myocytes." *J Appl Physiol 86* (2):584-91.

Palmer, B. M., A. M. Thayer, et al. (1998). "Shortening and [Ca2+] dynamics of left ventricular myocytes isolated from exercise-trained rats." *J Appl Physiol 85* (6):2159-68.

Park, Y., S. Kenekal, et al. (1992). "Oxidative changes in hypoxic rat heart tissue." *American Journal of Physiology* 260:H1395-H1405.

Powers, S. K., D. Criswell, et al. (1993). "Rigorous exercise training increases superoxide dismutase activity in ventricular myocardium." *Am J Physiol 265* (6 Pt 2):H2094-8.

Ramires, P. R. and L. L. Ji (2001). "Glutathione supplementation and training increases myocardial resistance to ischemia-reperfusion in vivo." *Am J Physiol Heart Circ Physiol 281* (2):H679-88.

Schaible, T. and J. Scheuer (1985). "Cardiac adaptations to chronic exercise." *Progress in Cardiovascular Disease* 27:297-324.

Seiler, K. S., J. P. Kehrer, et al. (1996). "Exogenous glutathione attenuates stunning following intermittenthypoxia in isolated rat hearts." *Free Radical Research 24* (2):115-22.

Simpson, P. J. and B. R. Lucchesi (1987). "Free radicals and myocardial ischemia and reperfusion injury." *Journal of Laboratory and Clinical Medicine* 110:13-30.

Singh, A., K. J. Lee, et al. (1989). "Relation between myocardial glutathione content and extent of ischemia- reperfusion injury." *Circulation 80* (6):1795-804.

Sochman, J., J. Vrbska, et al. (1996). "Infarct Size Limitation: acute N-acetylcysteine defense (ISLAND trial): preliminary analysis and report after the first 30 patients." *Clin Cardiol 19* (2):94-100.

Spencer, R. G., P. M. Buttrick, et al. (1997). "Function and bioenergetics in isolated perfused trained rat hearts." *Am J Physiol 272* (1 Pt 2):H409-17.

Symons, J. D., S. V. Rendig, et al. (2000). "Microvascular and myocardial contractile responses to ischemia: influence of exercise training." *J Appl Physiol 88* (2):433-42.

Tang, L. D., J. Z. Sun, et al. (1991). "Beneficial effects of N-acetylcysteine and cysteine in stunned myocardium in perfused rat heart." *Br J Pharmacol 102* (3):601-6.

Tani, M., Y. Suganuma, et al. (1997). "Decrease in ischemic tolerance with aging in isolated perfused Fischer 344 rat hearts: relation to increases in intracellular Na+ after ischemia." *J Mol Cell Cardiol 29* (11):3081-9.

Tsan, M. F., J. E. White, et al. (1989). "Modulation of endothelial GSH concentrations: effect of exogenous GSH and GSH monoethyl ester." *Journal of Applied Physiology 66* (3):1029-34.

Turan, B., M. Desilets, et al. (1996). "Oxidative effects of selenite on rat ventricular contractility and Ca movements." *Cardiovasc Res 32* (2):351-61.

Verbunt, R. J., W. G. Van Dockum, et al. (1996). "Postischemic injury in isolated rat hearts is not aggravated by prior depletion of myocardial glutathione." *Mol Cell Biochem 156* (1):79-85.

Wang, P. and J. L. Zweier (1996). "Measurement of nitric oxide and peroxynitrite generation in the postischemic heart. Evidence for peroxynitrite-mediated reperfusion injury." *J Biol Chem 271* (46):29223-30.

Werns, S. W., J. C. Fantone, et al. (1992). "Myocardial glutathione depletion impairs recovery of isolated blood- perfused hearts after global ischaemia." *J Mol Cell Cardiol 24* (11):1215-20.

Zweier, J. L., P. Kuppusamy, et al. (1988). "Measurement of endothelial cell free radical generation: evidence for a central mechanism of free radical injury in postischemic tissues." *Proc Natl Acad Sci USA 85* (11):4046-50.

Exercise and Immune System-related Diseases

RYOICHI NAGATOMI

Department of Medicine & Science in Sports & Exercise,
Tohoku University Graduate School of Medicine, Sendai, Japan.

Correspondence to:

Ryoichi Nagatomi MD & PhD
Tohoku University Graduate School of Medicine
Seiryo-machi 2-1, Aoba-ku,
Sendai 980-8575 Japan
Tel/Fax: +81-22-717-7768
E-mail: natagatomi@mail.cc.tohoku.ac.jp

Summary

Although recent advances in immunology brought us a better understanding of the pathophysiology of immune system-related diseases, such as autoimmune disease or allergic disease, we only have a limited amount of information on how disease activity is influenced by physical exercise. Although physical exercise involves a constellation of transient changes in the immune system, exercise intervention studies of patients with rheumatoid arthritis, systemic lupus erythematosus, multiple sclerosis, or bronchial asthma show negligible influence on the immunopathogenesis of these diseases within a moderate range of exercise intensity and duration. However, considering the various beneficial effects of exercise on autoimmune disease that the patients revealed during the intervention studies, such as reduction in joint pain, enhancement in functional capacity, avoidance of deconditioning, or the improvement in aerobic capacity, a tolerated level of exercise is recommendable. Exercise seems also favorable for HIV infected patients not only by avoiding muscle atrophy, but also by somewhat postponing the reduction of peripheral blood CD4 T cell counts reflecting the disease activity. Exercise may have a relatively small potential to affect the disease once it is established, but considering the health benefits of exercise, physical exercise is recommendable to the majority of patients with immune-related diseases with certain precautions.

1   Introduction

In clinical practice, when doctors give advice to their patients regarding their every day life, it is best advised to give them information based on epidemiological evidence. Yet in general, we have poor evidence as to how a patient with diseases due to a failure or dysregulation of the immune system should deal with their daily physical activity. Is it safe to exercise? Is physical activity favorable or unfavorable to the disease?

Modern immunology, as well as other fields of biological science, have made tremendous progress in the past decade thanks to the development of genetical analysis and manipulation. Recent advances in immunology revealed that the components of the immune system, as well as those of other systems have to a large extent to overlapping roles. Therefore, it is no exaggeration to say that components of the immune system are involved in a great majority of diseases we experience. Because it is difficult to cover all the immunological involvement, diseases caused presumably by failures or dysregulation of the immune system, and by pathological agents that mainly elicit immune responses as the major event of pathogenesis, will be focused on in this chapter. The disease category discussed will be autoimmune diseases, allergic diseases, and infectious diseases.

Physical exercise is known to elicit various changes in the immune system in both an acute and chronic manner. The moderate amount and intensity of exercise are generally accepted to bring either no change or a change that seems favorable, whereas long lasting and strenuous exercise are considered to be immunosuppressive for a certain period of time even after the exercise. Precise mechanisms that account for the changes related to exercise are still unknown. The changes in the components of the immune system during or after exercise may be caused in part as a general response to stress, however, tissue damage such as muscle injury may complicate the outcome. To date, whether exercise could specifically cause any significant change in the immune system during and after exercise is still a question to be answered. Moreover, there is only a small number of experimental evidence that would allow us to understand the biological significance of the changes brought about by exercise.

In this chapter, the immune system will briefly be overviewed to remind readers of the components of the immune system, in order to help with the understanding of the mechanism underlying the development of immune related diseases. Thereafter, the mechanism involving the pathogenesis of each immune disease will be discussed. Finally, epidemiological studies will be referred to, and discussed as to understand the influence of exercise on the course of each immune-related disease.

2 Brief Overview of the Immune System (Janeway and Travers 1997)

The immune system has a variety of effector systems to eliminate intruding pathogenic microbes and tumors. The innate immune system, which targets certain non-self structures, confronts microbes in the early phase of infection. The self structure of cells is usually protected from the innate immune system by inhibiting the activation of trigger responses of the innate immunity. The innate immune system usually acts in a non-amplifying manner as compared to the adaptive immune system that has a potential to respond to virtually all non-self substances, and microbes that a man should encounter in his life. An adaptive immune response to microbes on its first encounter usually involves a small number of cells. In several days, the number of cells able to react specifically to the microbes will be greatly amplified to an extent sufficient enough to confront the microbes. After the initiation of an adaptive immune response against infecting microbes, components of innate immunity and adaptive immune response may work in a co-operative manner that would eliminate the microbes more efficiently.

a) Cytokines

Cytokines are proteins produced and secreted by cells that modify the function of other cells by binding to cytokine receptors specific for each cytokine. Those mainly secreted by lymphocytes are termed lymphokines or interleukins (IL) followed by numbers which originally represented the order of discovery. Many cytokines are termed according to their function, such as tumor necrosis factor (TNF), interferon (IFN), transforming growth factor (TGF), and so on. Chemokines are a group of cytokines that trigger cell motility; they are important for the migration and activation of lymphocytes and phagocytes in immune responses. Cytokines have multiple functions. Cytokines such as IL-10, TGF beta are known as anti-inflammatory, and have a potent inhibitory effect on cellular functions, but would also induce differentiation of target cells.

b) Innate immune system

The innate immune system comprises various cellular components and effector proteins, the function of which do not necessarily depend upon antigen recognition. The innate immune system readily reacts against intruding microbes and altered cells of its own, but generally lacks an adaptive amplification procedure as typically seen with T and B lymphocytes. Some components of the innate immune system can also be activated by adaptive immune response, and contribute to the elimination of pathogens co-operatively.

I Complements

Complements are a group of plasma proteins that get fixed either to bacterial cell surfaces or to IgG or IgM antibodies bound to cell surfaces. Fixation leads to enzymatic activation of compliment proteins finally to form membrane-attack complexes that destroy the cell by boring holes on the cell membrane. During the activation procedure, several cleaved fragment s of complement proteins serve as chemoattractant to recruit phagocytes at the site of activation. Fixed complement proteins also facilitate phagocytes to ingest the cell by linking it to complement receptors of phagocytes, a process known as opsonization.

II Phagocytes

Phagocytes are cellular components characterized by their ability to ingest particulate matter such as bacteria. Ingested bacteria are usually destroyed by the exposure to lysosomal enzymes. The major phagocytes are neutrophils, monocytes, monocyte-derived macrophages, and tissue macrophages.

Neutrophils have the highest bactericidal potential due to their high content of lysosomal enzymes. The lack of neutrophil function as typically seen in patients with chronic granulomatous disease leads to recurrent bacterial infection. Release of lysosomal enzymes and production of oxygen radicals by neutrophils may often lead to tissue damage.

Monocytes leave the bone marrow moving into circulation, and finally lodge in various tissues where they differentiate into macrophages. There is a distinct population of macrophages called tissue macrophages such as alveolar macrophages or Kupffer cells of the liver. Tissue macrophages are thought to renew in situ. Macrophages usually have lower bactericidal activity, but inflammatory cytokines such as IFN gamma greatly enhance their potential. Macrophages are also characterized by their antigen presenting and co-stimulatory functions required for lymphocyte activation in adaptive immunity.

Monocytes are also known to develop into dendritic cells which do not have phagocytic activity but have strong antigen presenting and co-stimulatory functions. Because dendritic cells lack phagocytic ability, the antigens they present to lymphocytes are mainly viruses and chemical substances that enter the cells without being phagocytized.

III Natural killer cells

Natural killer (NK) cells are a subset of lymphocytes with no T or B lymphocyte markers rich in intracellular granules. They lack antigen receptors, and most of them lack both T and B cell markers. Recently, CD3 positive NK cells, known as NKT cells, were discovered. While NK cells produce IFN gamma, NKT cells produce IL-4. Both NK and NKT cells destroy cells bearing modified or altered major histocompatibility complex (MHC). They may destroy certain tumor cells and virus-infected cells. Patients who lack NK cells are known to suffer from severe herpes simplex or cytomegalo virus infection, but not from upper respiratory tract infection or bacterial infection. Because NK and NKT cells produce IFN gamma or IL-4, they may influence the differentiation of naïve T cells upon antigen recognition.

IV Gamma delta T cells

A subset of T cells that bear a gamma:delta heterodimeric T cell receptor unlike the common T cells bearing an alpha:beta heterodimeric T cell receptor chain has a narrow antigen specificity, possibly to recognize self antigens such as a heat shock protein. They may also be important in the early phase of bacterial infection.

c) Adaptive immune system

I Antibody

Antibody proteins are plasma proteins collectively called immunoglobulins produced by plasma cells differentiated from B lymphocytes upon antigen presentation at secondary lymphoid organs. They bind specifically to antigens, thereby blocking pathogens to enter cells or prepare them to be ingested and destroyed by phagocytes. There are 5 subtypes of immunoglobulins; IgG, IgM, IgA, IgE and IgD. IgM and IgG are the major immunoglobulins in the blood stream. IgM is generally produced in the early phase of infection, whereas IgG is produced in the later phase of infection, and maintained in the blood stream for a longer time of period avoiding infection of the same pathogen. Inactivated viruses, viral antigenic components, or inactivated bacterial toxins can deliberately be given to induce antigen specific IgG for protection against infection of particular pathogens. This procedure is well known as vaccination. IgG and IgM, when bound to cells bearing antigens, can fix and activate complements, which lead finally to the destruction of the cell. IgA forms a dimeric complex, and is secreted into the luminal surface of the mucous membrane. Specific IgA gives protection against particular pathogens such as viruses.

II Lymphocytes

B lymphocytes bear IgM as antigenic receptors on their surface. Upon conjugation of antigenic structures, they differentiate into plasma cells to produce specific antibodies. They also serve as an antigen presenting cell to T cells. Bound antigen will be internalized, and processed antigenic fragments will be conjugated to major histocompatibility complexes (MHC) which stimulate T cells specific for the particular antigen together with co-stimulatory molecules.

T lymphocytes mature in the thymus gland. The thymus not only harbors and helps T lymphocytes mature, but also eliminates auto-reactive T cells, by inducing, apoptosis. T lymphocytes have various subsets each having distinct roles. Those expressing CD4 are known as helper T cells, and are further divided into functional subsets according to the type of cytokines they produce. CD4 T cells that produce macrophage activating cytokines such as IFN gamma are known as Th1 cells. Th1 cells are specialized for activation and regulation of macrophages that are infected by or have ingested pathogenic microbes. CD4 T cells that produce cytokines that activate B cells, such as IL-4, IL-5, IL-6 and IL-10 are known as Th2 cells. Th2 cells are specialized for activating and regulating B cells to develop humoral immunity. The recognition of non-self in the adaptive immune response is based on a small structure of non-self substances or microbes termed antigens. Interestingly, Th1 and Th2 cells antagonize each other through production of their specific cytokines. Interferon gamma produced by Th1 or NK cells, and IL-12, which is produced by macrophages upon activation by IFN gamma, prohibit naïve cells (Th0) that have not yet encountered antigens into Th2 type cells and promote differentiation into Th1 type. On the contrary, IL-4, IL-5, and IL-10 all inhibit Th0 from differentiating into Th1 type. Interleukin-10 is a potent inhibitor of macrophage function, facilitating Th2 differentiation. Those expressing CD8 are known as cytotoxic T cells that can selectively kill cells bearing specific antigens by inducing apoptosis. CD8 cells kill virus-infected cells presenting viral antigens on their MHC class I molecule, and deprive the viruses of the site of replication. CD8 cells are essential for the elimination of infected viruses. Incomplete elimination of viruses by CD8 cells leads to persistent infection, such as chronic viral hepatitis.

3 Autoimmune Diseases

A. Immunopathogenesis of autoimmune diseases

Autoimmune disease is characterized by a specific adaptive immune response against self antigens. Because self antigens cannot be eliminated completely, the immune effector mechanism attacks the tissues that express the antigens persistently to cause a chronic disease. Autoimmune diseases can be classified by the immunopathogenic mechanisms being involved as in hypersensitivity diseases. The classification largely depends upon the location, and the type of self-antigens being targeted, and the effector components involved (Table 1).

Table 1

Type of disease	Self Antigen	Effector components	Example
IgG antibody mediated	Cell- or matrix-associated	IgG antibody, anemia, complement, phagocyte	Autoimmune hemolytic acute rheumatic fever, Goodpasture's syndrome
Immune-complex	Soluble antigen	IgG antibody, complement, phagocyte	Systemic lupus erythematosus (SLE)
T cell mediated	Cell-associated	CD4+ T cell, CD8+ Tcell phagocyte	Rheumatoid arthritis, multiple sclerosis, type I diabetes

The first category of autoimmune diseases is characterized by the production of IgG antibodies against cell surface or extracellular matrix anigens. Antibody binding leads to the destruction of the targeted cells or tissues by the activation of either a complement system, or phagocytes, or both. In autoimmune hemolytic anemia, an antibody binding to a Rh blood group antigen of red blood cells destroys the red blood cells leading to anemia. A cross reaction of antibodies raised against a bacterial cell wall antigen to the cardiac muscle component leads to myocarditis and scar formation at the cardiac valves in rheumatic fever. Goodpasture's syndrome is characterized by glomerulonephritis due to antibodies against the glomerular basement membrane.

The second category is characterized by the complement and phagocyte activation against deposited immune complexes at vascular walls. In systemic lupus erythematosus, autoantibodies directed at intracellular nucleoproteins common for virtually all cells of the body bind the antigens released from the cells to form a large amount of immune complexes. They are deposited at the vascular walls of small blood vessels, such as in the renal glomeruli and joints.

The third category is characterized by the activation of an autoreactive T cell-mediated effector mechanism against cell surface antigens. In rheumatoid arthritis (RA), components of joint synovial membrane are supposed to be recognized by autoreactive Th1 cells, which may trigger local inflammation by secreting inflammatory cytokines involving granulocytes and macrophages. Multiple sclerosis is another example in which the myelin basic protein of the neuronal sheath is supposed to be the antigen recognized. Cytotoxic CD8 T cells can also target and destroy self organs as in insulin dependent diabetes mellitus (type I diabetes). Although the susceptibility to autoimmune diseases is known to depend largely upon one's genetic background, one might assume physical stress may affect the progression of autoimmune diseases if physical exercise has a considerable impact on a particular fork of the immune system that involves the pathogenesis of autoimmune diseases mentioned above.

B. Effect of exercise on autoimmune diseases

There are only a limited number of studies that focused on the influence of physical exercise on autoimmune diseases from an immunological point of view. Among the wide variety of autoimmune diseases, those that severely interfere with physical activity because of joint inflammation such as RA or SLE have attracted the attention of investigators concerning the effect of physiotherapy including exercise.

1. Rheumatoid arthritis

The consequences of certain levels of physical activity or exercise intervention would give some insight into the effect, if any, of physical exercise on the inflammatory fork of the immune system that attacks the joint tissues in RA.

Stenstrom followed 69 non-hospitalized, functionally independent patients with RA for 4 years, and found out that the level of radiological progression of joint destruction correlated with the erythrocyte sedimentation rate, but not with the exercise frequency (Stenstrom 1994). A long term observation of 23 patients with RA, who were given physical training of various types for 4 to 8 years, revealed a slower progression of joint destruction in the trained patients as compared with control patients without any exercise intervention (Nordemar, Ekblom et al. 1981). Similar to the observation studies, none of the intervention studies have reported any deleterious effects of exercise training on disease activity of RA, such as joint pain or swelling, irrespective of the type of exercise employed (Karten, Lee et al. 1973; Daltroy, Robb-Nicholson et al. 1995; Harkcom, Lampman et al. 1985; Hoenig, Groff et al. 1993; van den Ende, Hazes et al. 1996; Komatireddy, Leitch et al. 1997; Bostrom, Harms-Ringdahl et al. 1998; Klepper 1999; McMeeken, Stillman et al. 1999).

Various modes of exercise were shown even to improve joint symptoms, such as aerobic exercise (Harkcom, Lampman et al. 1985; Klepper 1999), resistance exercise (Komatireddy, Leitch et al. 1997), and exercise therapy intended to increase the range of motion of specific joints, such as hand or knee (Hoenig, Groff et al. 1993; McMeeken, Stillman et al. 1999). Effectiveness of exercise training on various functional capacity measurements, such as aerobic capacity and muscle strength of RA patients, differs depending on the type of exercise performed as would be expected in the healthy population. Resistance type of strength training improves muscle strength (Hakkinen, Malkia et al. 1997; Komatireddy, Leitch et al. 1997); whereas aerobic type of exercise improves mainly cardiovascular fitness (Karten, Lee et al. 1973; Harkcom, Lampman et al. 1985; van den Ende, Hazes et al. 1996; Klepper 1999). The duration of training of the above studies ranged from 6 weeks to 6 months. But it seems to be important to maintain the exercise habit to prevent, or minimize the loss of physical capacity in RA because the discontinuation of exercise was shown to lead to a quick loss of the gain in physical capacity achieved by training (Van den Ende, Hazes et al. 1996; Hakkinen, Malkia et al. 1997). As for the epidemiological quality of the studies, a meta-analytical study by Van den Ende could select 6 randomized control trials among 30 controlled trials with aerobic exercise intervention for RA patients. None of the studies were detrimental to disease activity and joint pain, and they were effective in increasing aerobic capacity and muscle strength, but because of the heterogeneity in the outcome measures, the long term effect of dynamic or aerobic exercise on disease activity could not be assessed (Van den Ende, Vliet Vlieland et al. 1998).

Thus, classical physiotherapy intended to increase articular range of motion, aerobic exercise of moderate intensity, and resistive exercise all seem to bring little or no significant impact on the immune system that could affect the disease activity of RA. Clinical trials in which the effect of moderate exercise on RA related immunological measures were determined to show little influence of physical exercise on RA immunity. Rheumatoid factor, an immune complex (IC) of IgG and IgM anti IgG, is known to be involved in the joint destruction in co-operation with the complement system. Petersen et al. found no influence of exercise on RA patients compared to bed rest on the circadian change of the level of serum immune complex and complement activity (Petersen, Baatrup et al. 1986). Rall showed no effect of 12 weeks of high intensity progressive resistance training on PBMC subsets, serum levels of interleukin (IL)-1 beta, tumor necrosis factor-alpha (TNF), IL-6 and IL-2, or PGE2 production, lymphocyte proliferation, or DTH response (Rall, Roubenoff et al. 1996). Baslund reported the effects of 8 weeks progressive bicycle training , which resulted in the increase in maximal oxygen consumption on immune parameters, and found no significant change in serum levels of IL-1alpha and beta, IL-6, PBMC subsets and proliferative response, and NK cell activity before and after training(Baslund, Lyngberg et al. 1993).

Most of the above exercise studies dealt with patients who were classified into class I, II, or III of the functional categories proposed by the American Rheumatism Association (Hochberg, Chang et al. 1992). Recently patients even in class IV, almost incapable of carrying out even self-care tasks because of severe joint destruction and inflammation, were shown to be effectively treated to allow remarkable improvement in the joint inflammation, so that substantial numbers of patients could be re-categorized into a higher functional category by blockage of pro-inflammatory cytokines TNF or IL-6 (Feldmann and Maini 2001; Yoshizaki, Nishimoto et al. 1998). The therapeutic effect of blocking TNF alpha or IL-6 on joint inflammation of RA suggests direct involvement of these cytokines in the progression of RA.

Conditions that lead to an increase in the levels of these cytokines in the joints may well aggravate inflammation. In strenuous exercise, such as marathon and triathlon races, it is well known that the levels of proinflammatory cytokines increase (Northoff and Berg 1991; Northoff, Weinstock et al. 1994). A transient rise in the serum level of TNFalpha was detected after a competitive 5km road race (Espersen, Elbaek et al. 1990). The increase in the level of serum IL-6 was detected after a marathon race (Suzuki, Yamada et al. 2000). An elevation in serum IL-6 levels was also detected after repeated concentric contraction of an identical workload, suggesting the role of muscle damage in the induction of IL-6 (Bruunsgaard, Galbo et al. 1997). Prolonged submaximal eccentric exercise also results in the elevation of serum IL-6 levels (Rohde, MacLean et al. 1997). Elevation in the serum levels of both TNF alpha and IL-6 was found after strenuous circuit training (Brenner, Natale et al. 1999), exhaustive running exercise (Weinstock, Konig et al. 1997), and after a marathon race (Camus, Poortmans et al. 1997). It is not established whether a transient rise in serum pro-inflammatory cytokines, as observed after strenuous exercise, could actually affect the autoimmune process of RA, but considering the remote effect of these cytokines to promote acute phase inflammatory response, it wouldn't be a wise choice to take the risk. It is shown that in the synovial fluid of the exercising joint of RA patients, the activity of alpha 1-antitrypsin (alpha 1-AT), a potent physiological serine protease inhibitor, is markedly decreased without any change in the molecular form or quantitiy of alpha 1 AT. It is postulated that because alpha 1-AT is quickly inactivated when oxidized by a reactive oxygen species, a hypoxic-reperfusion injury after exercise may account for the marked reduction in joint alpha 1-AT activity. Thus, the potential for limiting inflammation, especially of complement activation, could be reduced in the exercising joint of RA patients (Zhang, Farrell et al. 1993).

In summary, both aerobic and strength training seem to be well tolerated by RA patients of class 1,2 and 3 as long as the intensity of exercise is moderate. The tolerated level of exercise training may well be beneficial, reducing joint pain and enhancing functional capacity. The impact of physical exercise on the inflammatory fork of the immune system responsible for RA pathogenesis seems to be negligible, as long as the intensity and duration is moderate. Although we lack clinical data, strenuous exercise that may accompany acute phase response possibly due to muscle damage, can aggravate joint inflammation.

2. Systemic Lupus Erythematosus (SLE)

Both SLE and RA have been classified as collagen diseases, and joint inflammation in both diseases was thought to be of a similar pathogenesis. As mentioned before, recent advances in immunology revealed that T helper cells targeted at unknown synovial proteins induce an inflammatory process that leads to joint destruction, whereas systemic precipitation of immune complexes on vascular walls triggers complement activation in SLE, which recruits inflammatory cells to cause vasculitis. Vasculitis that involves arterioles at the joint tissue is manifested as arthritis.

Unlike RA, in which inflammation is commonly localized at joints, any tissue can be affected in SLE patients because of vasculitis. While arthritis and glomerulonephritis are common in SLE, the lungs, brain and heart can also be affected. The incidence of abnormal myocardial perfusion in patients with SLE is relatively high, exceeding one-third of randomly selected patients (Hosenpud, Montanaro et al. 1984). Even asymptomatic children, when examined by radionuclide imaging, might be predisposed to the early-onset ischemic heart disease in adult SLE patients (Gazarian, Feldman et al. 1998). Exercise tests also revealed an abnormal left ventricular function in more than one third of the patients examined (Bahl, Aradhye et al. 1992). The incidence of cardiac valvular disorder, angina, and electrocardiographic ischemic pattern both at rest and during exercise in SLE patients, was accordingly high in a larger scale study in Sweden (Sturfelt, Eskilsson et al. 1992). Pulmonary arterial pressure is higher in SLE patients, both at rest and during exercise which may largely contribute to reduced exercise, capacity in patients with SLE (Winslow, Ossipov et al. 1993). Thus, while the exercise capacity of patients with RA may be limited principally due to musculoskeletal disorder, that of patients with SLE may be limited due to cardiovascular problems. A patient with SLE may have little problem in a sedentary life, but a certain level of exercise might endanger his life when myocardial oxygen demand exceeds its supply. It is, therefore, especially important for patients with SLE to have their cardiac and pulmonary function examined intensively when they wish to be engaged in a regular exercise program or sports activity.

How can regular exercise influence the disease activity of SLE for those patients who can tolerate exercise from a cardiological point of view? An 8-week aerobic conditioning program for patients with SLE was shown to increase their aerobic capacity without exacerbating the disease (Robb-Nicholson, Daltroy et al. 1989). Six months of minimally supervised home aerobic exercise was shown to be safe without any exacerbation of SLE and RA in a randomized controlled trial (Daltroy, Robb-Nicholson et al. 1995). A cross sectional analysis of 100 women with SLE showed no significant association of exercise frequency with morbidity in SLE, such as physical disability, disease activity, and organ damage (Ward, Lotstein et al. 1999). Although the number of studies is limited, moderate amount and intensity of exercise have little effect on the immune mechanism underlying SLE, as well as in RA.

Immune complexes are the major pathogenic component of SLE. The major antigenic components of ICs in SLE are intracellular nucleoproteins that are present in virtually all cellular components of the body. Destruction of any cells may result in the release of otherwise hidden nucleoproteins that contributes to the formation of IC. These IC may aggravate the disease. A circulating amount of IC is known to fluctuate by various factors in healthy subjects, but the contribution of exercise to IC fluctuation in SLE is not established (Isenberg, Crisp et al. 1981; Simpson, Myles et al. 1983). Few clinical studies have dealt with the effect of strenuous exercise on circulating IC fluctuation, but considering the possible damage in muscle cells, it is best advised for the patients with SLE to refrain from heavy strenuous exercise. In an experimental rabbit model of IC mediated glomerulonephritis, 4 weeks of treadmill exercise was shown to aggravate the disease (Cornacoff, Hebert et al. 1985). The IC in this rabbit model of glomerulonephritis, however, is produced by a repeated injection of bovine serum albumin, and no measures associated with muscle destruction were evaluated in this study. The effect of exercise on circulating IC in association with tissue damage needs to be elucidated.

In summary, exercise, unless its intensity and amount are not high, may not affect the disease activity in SLE as well as in RA. Because of possible complication of coronary and pulmonary arteries, an appropriate exercise tolerance test should be carried out for patients with SLE before prescribing exercise.

4   Multiple sclerosis

In multiple sclerosis (MS), autoreactive T cells targeted at myelin related proteins in the central nervous system (CNS), such as myelin basic protein, mediate inflammatory changes in the CNS (Pender et al 1996; Wucherpfennig et al 1997; Krogsgaard et al 2000; Hellings et al 2001). Autoantibodies against myelin related proteins, together with complement activation, may also involve in the pathophysiology in some cases, and in some cases, viral infection instead of autoimmunity, may trigger the disease (Lucchinetti et al 2000). Because oligodendrocytes, which are responsible for maintenance of myelination of axons in the CNS (Keirstead et al 1999), express a large amount of myelin related proteins, the attack by autoreactive T cells leads to demyelination, which affects saltatory conduction in the CNS. Because demyelination may take place anywhere in the CNS, patients with MS suffer a wide variety of symptoms, which vary from patient to patient. A common synptom among most of the patients with MS is the exacerbation of CNS symptoms when exposed to heat, or during physical exercise. Exacerbation of CNS symptoms induced by exercise may be due to the heat produced by muscle activity, because the cooling of lower extremities before 30 min. of exercise of moderate intensity significantly improved walk performance, and reduced the perceived rating of exertion (White et al 2000). Increased body temperature is thought to increase ionic conduction and reduce the duration of the action potential. This reduces the amount of current resulting in the slowing of the conduction speed and/or the conduction block (Guthrie et al 1995). Dysautonomia further impairs the thermoregulation during exercise (Noronha et al 1968). Therefore, exercise-induced exacerbation of MS is not likely to be because of the impact of exercise on the immune system.

Serve fatigue, which affects about 85% of MS patients (Krupp te al 1988), is one of the major causes of withdrawing patients with MS from regular physical activity. Because the reduction in daily physical activity results in further deconditioning of the musculoskeletal system, a balance between regular physical activity and rest is preferred to immobility in order to reduce fatigue and deconditioning (Freal et al 1984).

A randomized controlled trial to assess the effect of a 15 week-aerobic exercise intervention for MS patients resulted in a significant improvement in fitness measures, and a positive impact on factors related to the quality of life such as POMS, depression, and anger scores in the exercise group without increasing the incidence of exacerbations (Petajan et al 1996).

In summary, although MS largely interferes with patients' physical performance, regular exercise is preferred to avoid immobility and deconditioning, provided that a rise in the body temperature is carefully controlled. The impact of exercise intervention on the responsible immunoppathogenesis of MS seems to be negligible.

5 Allergic Disease

A. Immunopathogenesis of allergic diseases

Allergic diseases are characterized by an adaptive immune response against extrinsic innocuous antigens that lead to IgE production. The causative antigens are not always identified, but a majority of them are thought to be common in the environment where the patients live. While food allergies and systemic anaphylaxis may manifest systemic and acute symptoms often life-threatening, repeated antigen exposure to the airway may lead to chronic diseases. Secreted IgE cause mast cell degranulation which causes a wide variety of diseases depending on the site of antigen entry (Table 2).

Table 2

Disease	Site of entry	Symptom and findings
Bronchial asthma	Lower respiratory tract	Bronchospasm Edema of airway mucosa
Allergic rhinitis	Upper respiratory tract	Nasal discharge and irritation Edema of nasal mucosa
Food allergy	Intestine	Diarrhea Vomiting Urticaria
Anaphylaxis	Blood stream	Circulatory collapse

Among the allergic diseases listed on the table, bronchial asthma is extensively investigated in relationship with exercise because it could critically affect the exercise performance.

B. Exercise induced asthma

The prevalence of bronchial asthma in athletes is remarkably high as compared to the prevalence in the normal population (Leuppi, Kuhn et al. 1998; Nystad, Harris et al. 2000). The prevalence tends to be higher in those engaged in strenuous exercise such as ice-hockey (Leuppi, Kuhn et al. 1998), and endurance exercise such as cross-country skiing (Nystad, Harris et al. 2000).

Exercise induced broncospasm is a common complication among asthmatic patients characterized by the transient narrowing of airway following vigorous exercise. The prevalence of exercise-induced asthma (EIA) is also higher in elite Olympic level athletes, who are engaged in endurance or strength types of exercise, such as cross-country skiing, cycling and moutain biking (Wilber, Rundell et al. 2000; Weiler, Layton et al. 1998).

As bronchial asthma may be caused by IgE mediated immune response to inhaled antigens such as pollen or house dust, an increase of the inflammatory cells is commonly detected in the airway epithelia in elite cross-country skiers, as well as in asthmatic patients (Sue-Chu, Larsson et al. 1999; Karjalainen, Laitinen et al. 2000). Eosinophil is a member of granulocytes which expresses higher levels of the IgE Fc receptor that mediates IgE hyperresponsiveness. Consequently, the severity of bronchoconstriction evoked by exercise was shown to be closely related to eosinophilic airway inflammation (Yoshikawa, Shoji et al. 1998). Mast cell activation was also shown to be involved in exercise induced bronchoconstriction (EIB) (O'Sullivan, Roquet et al. 1998).

At first, EIB was thought to be triggered by the cooling and warming of the airway epithelia resulting in hyperemia and edema of the epithelia. But because broncoconstriction was shown to occur without cooling and heating, it is now considered that dehydration of epithelia, due to a large increase in the passage of air during strenuous or endurance exercise, plays an essential role in EIB. Large amounts of air passage facilitates evaporation of water from the airway leading to dehydration, and shrinkage of the epithelial cells, that finally leads to the release of inflammatory mediators that trigger smooth muscle cell contraction (Anderson and Daviskas 2000).

It is possible to prevent EIB by avoiding vigorous exercise , but several exercise trials revealed a successful attempt in reducing EIB. Post-exercise broncoconstriction could be reduced by a brief warm-up exercise that reduced the drop in the peak flow rate (de Bisschop, Guenard et al. 1999). Six weeks of swimming as training for asthmatic children successfully improved their aerobic capacity, but failed to improve the airway hypersensitivity (Matsumoto, Araki et al. 1999). A systematic review by Ram cited 8 exercise trials for asthmatic patients, and found that despite the improvement in aerobic fitness, there was only a minimal change in the lung function (Ram, Robinson et al. 2000). Hallstrand was also successful in improving aerobic fitness of mild asthmatic patients (Hallstrand, Bates et al. 2000). Nonetheless, improvement in aerobic capacity, even without improvement in the airway sensitivity, may well benefit the asthmatic patients.

Thus, exercise induced asthma seems to be a state evoked, rather by the physiological nature of exercise, than by any immunological impact of exercise on the hypersensitivity mechanism. Exercise training seems to have neither significant influence on the hypersensitivity mechanism, such as IgE production, nor on degranulation of mast cells.

6 Human Immunodeficiency Virus Infection

Human Immunodeficiency Virus (HIV) is a causative agent for Acquired Immune Deficiency Syndrome (AIDS). HIV is an enveloped retrovirus that infects CD4 T cells and macrophages. CD4 serves as a virus receptor for HIV, and the chemokine receptor CXCR4 has also been shown to mediate infection of HIV. The extensive immunodeficiency syndrome characterized by opportunistic infection is caused by a substantial loss of CD4 T cells. CD4 T cells may be killed directly by the virus, killed through induction of apoptosis, or killed by HIV-specific CD8 cytotoxic T cells. The causative agents of opportunistic infection show the range of CD4 T cell protection in an uninfected physiological state. They are fungi, parasites, intracellular bacteria, and viruses such as *Herpes simplex virus, Cytomegalovirus* and *Varicella zoster virus*. HIV is also known to affect the central nervous system (CNS) leading to dementia and psychotic symptoms. Infected macrophages seem to be responsible for the spreading of the viruses to CNS. Infection to CNS may be one of the causes for systemic wasting syndrome typical in the later phase of AIDS. Abnormally elevated pro-inflammatory cytokines such as IL-6 and TNF alpha, may also be responsible for extensive muscle wasting in AIDS.

Muscle wasting and depression quickly affect the quality of a patient's life. As a counter measure for wasting, exercise training has been employed (LaPerriere, Antoni et al. 1990; Elliot, Goldberg et al. 1992; Rigsby, Dishman et al. 1992; MacArthur, Levine et al. 1993). None have reported any deleterious effect on the course of reduction in CD4 T cells. A single bout of exercise was shown not to increase the viral load in the blood (Roubenoff, Skolnik et al. 1999). Later, aerobic exercise training was shown not only to prevent wasting, but also to prevent the loss of CD4 T cells from the blood stream (LaPerriere, Klimas et al.

1997). A cohort study, with an observation period of 6 years involving 159 HIV positive and 259 HIV negative homosexual individuals, also proved that moderate activity showed an increase in CD4 count, and a slower progression of the disease after 1 year (Mustafa, Sy et al. 1999). Unfortunately, after the 2nd year there was no statistical significance. Perna also reported the effect of a 12 week supervised exercise on pre-AIDS HIV positive patients, and found that CD 4 cell counts increased in the compliant exercisers (Perna, LaPerriere et al. 1999). To date a resistance exercise regimen in combination with androgen administration is shown to be effective in a larger gain of muscle mass, and increased physical capacity, without any deterioration in the disease activity (Strawford, Barbieri et al. 1999; Grinspoon, Corcoran et al. 2000).

The mechanism with which exercise slows or prevents the loss of CD4 T cells is still unknown, but exercise, both resistance and aerobic, are recommended for patients with HIV at least to expect a better quality of life.

7 Conclusion

Although there are a considerable number of reports regarding the alteration in the immune-related parameters after exercise, both acute and chronic, the effect of exercise on immune-related disease is relatively small. This does not mean that exercise does not affect the immune system, but it may arise because the specific fork of the immune system that involves the pathogenesis of immune-related disease was simply not influenced. Dramatic changes in the immune system after exercise are often shown using animal models, but these experiments mostly involve the effect of exercise in the early phase of disease onset. Patients with immune-related diseases have established diseases. We have less chance to deal with the onset of immune-related disease in patients when typical symptoms are not manifested. Exercise may have a relatively small potential to affect the disease once it is established, but considering the other health benefits, physical exercise is recommended to the majority of patients with immune-related diseases with certain precautions.

REFERENCES

Anderson, S. D. and E. Daviskas (2000). The mechanism of exercise-induced asthma is. *J Allergy Clin Immunol* **106**(3):453-9.

Bahl, V. K., Aradhye, R. S. Vasan, A. Malhotra, K. S. Reddy and A. N. Malaviya (1992). Myocardial systolic function in systemic lupus erythematosus: a study based on radionuclide ventriculography. *Clin Cardiol* **15**(6):433-5.

Baslund, B., K. Lyngberg, V. Andersen, J. Halkjaer Kristensen, M. Hansen, M. Klokker and B. K. Pedersen (1993). Effect of 8 weeks of bicycle training on the immune system of patients with rheumatoid arthritis. *J Appl Physiol* **75**(4): 1691-5.

Bostrom, C., K. Harms-Ringdahl, H. Karreskog and R. Nordemar (1998). Effects of static and dynamic shoulder rotator exercises in women with rheumatoid arthritis: a randomised comparison of impairment, disability, handicap, and health. *Scand J Rheumatol* **27**(4):281-90.

Brenner, I. K., V. M. Natale, P. Vasiliou, A. I. Moldoveanu, P. N. Shek and R. J. Shephard (1999). Impact of three different types of exercise on components of the inflammatory response. *Eur J Appl Physiol Occup Physiol* **80**(5):452-60.

Bruunsgaard, H., H. Galbo, J. Halkjaer-Kristensen (1997). Exercise-induced increase in serum interleukin-6 in humans is related to muscle damage. *J Physiol* **499**(Pt 3):833-41.

Camus, G., J. Poortmans, M. Nys, G. Deby-Dupont, J. Duchateau, C. Deby and M. Lamy (1997). Mild endotoxemia and the inflammatory response induced by a marathon race. *Clin Sci (Colch)* **92**(4):415-22.

Cornacoff, J. B., L. A. Herbert, H. M. Sharma, W. H. Bay and D. C. Young (1985). Adverse effect of exercise on immune complex-mediated glomerulonephritis. *Nephron* **40**(3):292-6.

Daltroy, L. H., C. Robb-Nicholson, M. D. Iversen, E. A. Wright and M. H. Liang (1995). Effectiveness of minimally supervised home aerobic training in patients with systemic rheumatic disease. *Br J Rheumatol* **34**(11):1064-9.

de Bisschop, C., H. Guenard, P. Desnot and J. Vergeret (1999). Reduction of exercise-induced asthma in children by short, repeated warm ups. *Br J Sports Med* 33(2):100-4.

Elliot, D. L., L. Goldberg and G. O. Coodley (1992). Physical conditioning among HIV-positive men. *Med Sci Sports Exerc* **24**(7):838-40.

Espersen, G. T., A. Elbaek, E. Ernst, E. Toft, S. Kaalund, C. Jersild and N. Grunnet (1990). Effect of physical exercise on cytokines and lymphocyte subpopulations in human peripheral blood. *Apmis* **98**(5):395-400.

Feldmann, M. and R. N. Maini (2001). ANTI-TNF{(alpha}} THERAPY OF RHEUMATOID ARTHRITIS: What Have We Learned? *Annu Rev Immunol* **19**: 163-196.

Gazarian, M., B. M. Feldman, L. N. Benson, D. L. Gilday, R. M. Laxer and E. D. Silverman (1998). Assessment of myocardial perfusion and function in childhood systemic lupus erythematosus. *J Pediatr* **132**(1): 109-16.

Grinspoon, S., C. Corcoran, K. Parlman, M. Costello, D. Rosenthal, E. Anderson, T. Stanley, D. Schoenfeld, B. Burrows, D. Hayden, N. Basgoz and A. Klibanski (2000). Effects of testosterone and progressive resistance training in eugonadal men with AIDS wasting. A randomized, controlled trial. *Ann Intern Med* **133**(5):348-55.

Hakkinen, A., E. Malkia, K. Hakkinen, I. Jappinen, L. Laitinen and P. Hannonen (1997). Effects of detraining subsequent to strength training on neuromuscular function in patients with inflammatory arthritis. *Br J Rheumatol* **36**(10):1075-81.

Hallstrand, T. S., P. W. Bates and R. B. Schoene (2000). Aerobic conditioning in mild asthma decreases the hyperpnea of exercise and improves exercise and ventilatory capacity. *Chest* **118**(5):1460-9.

Harkcom, T. M., R. M. Lampman, B. F. Banwell and C. W. Castor (1985). Therapeutic value of graded aerobic exercise training in rheumatoid arthritis. *Arthritis Rheum* **28**(1):32-9.

Hellings, N., M. Baree, C. Verhoeven, B. D'Hooghe M., R. Medaer, C. C. Bernard, J. Raus and P. Stinissen (2001). T-cell reactivity to multiple myelin antigens in multiple sclerosis patients and healthy controls. *J Neurosci Res* **63**(3):290-302.

Hochberg, M. C., R. W. Chang, I. Dwosh, S. Lindsey, T. Pincus and F. Wolfe (1992). The American College of Rheumatology 1991 revised criteria for the classification of global functional status in rheumatoid arthritis. *Arthritis Rheum* **35**(5):498-502.

Hoenig, H., G. Groff, K. Pratt, E. Goldberg and W. Franck (1993). A randomized controlled trial of home exercise on the rheumatoid hand. *J Rheumatol* **20**(5):785-9.

Hosenpud, J. D., A. Montanaro, M. V. Hart, J. E. Haines, H. D. Specht, R. M. Bennett and F. E. Kloster (1984). Myocardial perfusion abnormalities in asymptomatic patients with systemic lupus erythematosus. *Am J Med* **77**(2): 286-92.

Isenberg, D. A., A. J. Crisp, W. J. Morrow, D. Newham and M. L. Snaith (1981). Variation in circulating immune complex levels with diet, exercise, and sleep: a comparison between normal controls and patients with systemic lupus erythematosus. *Annals Of The Rheumatic Diseases* **40**(5):466-9.

Janeway, J. C. A. and P. Travers (1997). Immunobiology: the immune system in health and disease, Current Biology Ltd.

Karjalainen, E. M., A. Laitinen, M. Sue-Chu, A. Altraja, L. Bjermer and L. A. Laitinen (2000). Evidence of airway inflammation and remodeling in ski athletes with and without bronchial hyperresponsiveness to methacholine. *Am J Respir Crit Care Med* **161**(6):2086-91.

Karten, I., M. Lee and C. McEwen (1973). Rheumatoid arthritis: five-year study of rehabilitation. *Arch Phys Med Rehabil* **54**(3):120-8.

Keirstead, H. S. and W. F. Blakemore (1999). The role of oligodendrocytes and oligodendrocyte progenitors in CNS remyelination. *Adv Exp Med Biol* **468**: 183-97.

Klepper, S. E. (1999). Effects of an eight-week physical conditioning program on disease signs and symptoms in children with chronic arthritis. *Arthritis Care Res* **12**(1):52-60.

Komatireddy, G. R., R. W. Leitch, K. Cella, G. Browning and M. Minor (1997). Efficacy of low load resistive muscle training in patients with rheumatoid arthritis functional class II and III. *J Rheumatol* **24**(8):1531-9.

Krogsgaard, M., K. W. Wucherpfenning, B. Canella, B. E. Hansen, A. Svejgaard, J. Pyrdol, H. Ditzel, C. Raine, J. Engberg and L. Fugger (2000). Visualization of myelin basic protein (MBP) T cell epitopes in multiple sclerosis lesions using a monoclonal antibody specific for the human histocompatibility leukocyte antigen (HLA)-DR2-MBP 85-99 complex. *J. Exp Med* **191**(8):1395-412.

Krupp, L. B., A. Alvarez, N. G. La Rocca and L. C. Scheinberg (1988). Fatigue in multiple sclerosis. *Arch Neurol* **45**(4):435-7.

LaPerriere, A., N. Klimas, M. A. Fletcher, A. Perry, GO. Ironson, F. Perna and N. Schneiderman. Change in CD4+ cell enumeration following aerobic exercise training in HIV-1 disease: possible mechanisms and practical applications. *Int J Sports Med* **18 Suppl** 1:S56-61.

LaPerriere, A. R., M. H. Antoni, N. Schneiderman, G. Ironson, N. Klimas, P. Caralis and M. A. Fletcher (1990). Exercise intervention attenuates emotional distress and natural killer cell decrements following notification of positive serologic status for HIV-1. *Biofeedback Self Regul* **15**(3):229-42.

Leuppi, J. D., M. Kuhn, C. Comminot and W. H. Reinhart (1998). High prevalence of bronchial hyperresponsiveness and asthma in ice hockey players. *Eur Respir J* **12**(1):13-6.

Lucchinetti, C., W. Bruck, J. Parisi, B. Scheithauer, M. Rodriguez and H. Lassmann (2000). Heterogeneity of multiple sclerosis lesions: implications for the pathogenesis of demyelination. *Ann Neurol* **47**(6):707-17

MacArthur, R. D., S. D. Levine and T. J. Birk (1993). Supervised exercise training improves cardiopulmonary fitness in HIV-infected persons. *Med Sci Sports Exerc* **25**(6):684-8.

Matsumoto, I., H. Araki, K. Tsuda, H. Odajima, S. Nishima, Y. Higaki, H. Tanaka, M. Tanaka and M. Shindo (1999). Effects of swimming training on aerobic capacity and exercise induced bronchoconstriction in children with bronchial asthma. *Thorax* **54**(3):196-201.

McMeeken, J., B. Stillman, I. Story, P. Kent and Smith (1999). The effects of knee extensor and flexor muscle training on the timed-up- and-go test in individuals with rheumatoid arthritis. *Physiother Res Int* **4**(1):55-67.

Mustafa, T., F. S. Sy, C. A. Macera, S. J. Thompson, K. L. Jackson, A. Selassie and L. L. Dean (1999). Association between exercise and HIV disease progression in a cohort of homosexual men. *Ann Epidemiol* **9**(2):127-31.

Nordemar, R., B. Ekblom, L. Zachrisson and Lundqvist (1981). Physical training in rheumatoid arthritis: a controlled long-term study. I. *Scand J Rheumatol* **10**(1):17-23.

Northoff, H. and A. Berg (1991). Immunologic mediators as parameters of the reaction to strenuous exercise. *Int J Sports Med* **12 Suppl** 1:S9-15.

Northoff, H., C. Weinstock and A. Berg (1994). The cytokine response to strenuous exercise. *Int J Sports Med* **15 Suppl** 3:S167-71.

Nystad, W., J. Harris and J. S. Borgen (2000). Asthma and wheezing among Norwegian elite athletes. *Med Sci Sports Exerc* **32**(2):266-70.

O'Sullivan, S., A. Roquet, B. Dahlen, F. Larsen, A. Eklund, M. Kumlin, P. M. O'Byrne and S. E. Dahlen (1998). Evidence for mast cell activation during exercise-induced bronchoconstriction. *Eur Respir J* **12**(2):345-50.

Perna, F. M., P. A. Csurhes, R. A. Houghten, P. A. McCombe and M. F. Good (1999). Cardiopulmonary and CD4 cell changes in response to exercise training in early symptomatic HIV infection. *Med Sci Sports Exerc* **31**(7):973-9.

Petajan, J. H., E. Gappmaier, A. T. White, M. K. Spencer, L. Mino and R. W. Hicks (1986). Circadian and diurnal variation of circulating immune complexes, complement-mediated solubilization, and the complement split product C3d in rheumatoid arthritis. *Scand J Rheumatol* **15**(2):113-8.

Petersen, I., G. Baatrup, I. Brandslund, B. Teisner, G. G. Rasmussen and S. E. Svehag (1986). Circadian and diurnal variation of circulating immune complexes, complement-mediated solubilization, and the complement split product C3d in rheumatoid arthritis. *Scand J Rheumatol* **15**(2):113-8.

Rall, L. C., R. Roubenoff, J. G. Cannon, L. W. Abad, C. A. Dinarello and S. N. Meydani (1996). Effects of progressive resistance training on immune response in aging and chronic inflammation. *Med Sci Sports Exerc* **28**(11): 1356-65.

Ram, F. S., S. M. Robinson and P. N. Black (2000). Effects of physical training in asthma: a systematic review. *Br J Sports Med* **34**(3):162-7.

Rigsby, L. W., R. K. Dishman, A. W. Jackson, G. S. Maclean and P. B. Raven (1992). Effects of exercise training on men seropositive for the human immunodeficiency virus-1. *Med Sci Sports Exerc* **24**(1):6-12.

Robb-Nicholson, L. C., L. Daltroy, H. Eaton, V. Gall, E. Wright, L. H. Hartley, P. H. Schur and M. H. Liang (1989). Effects of aerobic conditioning in lupus fatigue: a pilot study. *Br J Rheumatol* **28**(6):500-5.

Rohde, T., D. A. MacLean, E. A. Richter, B. Kiens and B. K. Pedersen (1997). Prolonged submaximal eccentric exercise is associated with increased levels of plasma IL-6. *Am J Physiol* **273**(1 Pt 1):E85-91.

Roubenoff, R., P. R. Skolnik, A. Shevitz, L. Snydam, A. Wang, S. Melason and S. Gorbach (1999). Effect of a single bout of acute exercise on plasma human immunodeficiency virus RNA levels. *J Appl Physiol* **86**(4):1197-201.

Simpson, I. J., M. J. Myles and G. W. Smith (1983). Immune complexes in normal subjects. *Journal Of Clinical And Laboratory Immunology* **11**(3):119-22.

Stenstrom, C. H. (1994). Radiologically observed progression of joint destruction and its relationship with demographic factors, disease severity, and exercise frequency in patients with rheumatoid arthritis. *Phys Ther* **74**(1):32-9.

Strawford, A., T. Barbieri, M. Van Loan, E. Parks, D. Catlin, N. Barton, R. Neese, M. Christiansen, J. King and M. K. Hellerstein (1999). Resistance exercise and supraphysiologic androgen therapy in eugonadal men with HIV-related weight loss: a randomized controlled trial. *Jama* **281**(14):1282-90.

Sturfelt, G., J. Eskilsson, O. Nived, L. Truedsson and S. Valind (1992). Cardiovascular disease in systemic lupus erythematosus. A study of 75 patients form a defined population. *Medicine (Baltimore)* **71**(4):216-23.

Sue-Chu, M., L. Larsson, T. Moen, S. I. Rennard and L. Bjermer (1999). Bronchoscopy and bronchoalveolar lavage findings in cross-country skiers with and without "ski asthma" *Eur Respir J* **13**(3):626-32.

Suzuki, K., M. Yamada, S. Kurakake, N. Okamura, K. Yamaya, Q. Liu, S. Kudoh, K. Kowatari, S. Nakaji and K. Sugawara (2000). Circulating cytokines and hormones with immunosuppressive but neutrophil-priming potentials rise after endurance exercise in humans. *Eur J Appl Physiol* **81**(4):281-7.

Van den Ende, C. H., J. M. Hazes, S. le Cessie, W. J. Mulder, D. G. Belfor, F. C. Breedveld and B. A. Djikmans (1996). Comparison of high and low intensity training in well controlled rheumatoid arthritis. Results of a randomised clinical trial. *Ann Rheum Dis* **55**(11):798-805.

Van den Ende, C. H., T. P. Vliet Vlieland, M. Munneke and J. M. Hazes (1998). Dynamic exercise therapy in rheumatoid arthritis: a systematic review. *Br J Rheumatol* **37**(6):677-87.

Ward, M. M., D. S. Lotstein, T. M. Bush, R. E. Lambert, R. van Vollenhoven and C. M. Neuwelt (1999). Psychosocial correlates of morbidity in women with systemic lupus erythematosus. *J Rheumatol* **26**(10):2153-8.

Weiler, J. M., T. Layton and M. Hunt (1998). Asthma in United States Olympic athletes who participated in the 1996 Summer Games. *J Allergy Clin Immunol* **102**(5):722-6.

Weinstock, C., D. Konig, R. Harnischmacher, J. Keul, A. Berg and H. Northoff (1997). Effect of exhaustive exercise stress on the cytokine response. *Med Sci Sports Exerc* **29**(3):345-54.

Wilber, R. L., K. W. Rundell, L. Szmedra, D. M. Jenkinson, J. Im and S. D. Drake (2000). Incidence of exercise-induced bronchospasm in Olympic winter sport athletes. *Med Sci Sports Exerc* **32**(4):732-7.

Winslow, T. M., M. Ossipov, R. F. Redberg, G. P. Fazio and N. B. Schiller (1993). Exercise capacity and hemodynamics in systemic lupus erythematosus: a Doppler echocardiographic exercise study. *Am Heart J* **126**(2):410-4.

Wucherpfennig, K. W., I. Catz, S. Hausmann, J. L. Strominger, L. Steinman and K. G. Warren (1997). Recognition of the immunodominant myelin basic protein peptide by autoantibodies and HLA-DR2-restricted T cell clones from multiple sclerosis patients. Identity of key contact residues in the B-cell and T-cell epitopes. *J Clin Invest* **100**(5):1114-22.

Yoshikawa, T., S. Shoji, T. Fujii, H. Kanazawa, S. Kudoh, K. Hirata and J. Yoshikawa (1998). Severity of exercise-induced bronchoconstriction is related to airway eosinophilic inflammation in patients with asthma. *Eur Respir J* **12**(4):879-84.

Yoshizaki, K., N. Nishimoto, M. Mihara and T. Kishimoto (1998). Therapy of rheumatoid arthritis by blocking IL-6 signal transduction with a humanized anti-IL-6 receptor antibody. *Springer Semin Immunopathol* **20**(1-2):247-59.

Zhang, Z., A. J. Farell, D. R. Blake, K. Chidwick and P. G. Winyard (1993). Inactivation of synovial fluid alpha 1-antitrypsin by exercise of the inflamed rheumatoid joint. *FEBS Lett* **321**(2-3):274-8.

Exercise and Type 2 Diabetes Mellitus

SHUZO KUMAGAI

Institute of Health Science, Kyushu University, Kasuga, Fukuoka, Japan

Correspondence to:

Shuzo Kumagai Ph.D.
Institute of Health Science, Kyushu University, Kasuga, Fukuoka, Japan
E-mail: shuzo@ihs.kyushu-u.ac.jp

Summary

In this short review, we focused on the relationship between physical activity or physical fitness with glucose homeostasis in humans, subjects included healthy subjects and patients with diabetes mellitus. Most of the prospective cohort studies have consistently demonstrated there to be a lower relative risk or odds ratio in the population with higher physical activity and cardiorespiratory fitness. Randomized control trials suggest that the combination of diet and exercise therapy are the most useful treatments for the improvement of glucose homeostasis. The mechanism underlying increased insulin sensitivity after acute and chronic exercise was discussed. In addition, the effect of physical inactivity, and of exercise training on insulin resistance syndrome, and the effect of skeletal muscle profiles (i.e. fiber composition, enzyme activity and capillarization) on insulin resistance are also discussed. Finally, a psychological approach to maintain compliance with the health programs for treatment of obesity and Type 2 diabetes was proposed.

1 Introduction

Diabetes mellitus is the most common disease in developed countries, even in Japan. It is also a major risk factor for coronary heart disease (CHD), which is one of the endpoints caused by the natural course of diabetes mellitus. According to a recent epidemiological survey in Japan, the prevalence rates were averaged at 22.8% for impaired glucose tolerance (IGT) and 10.0% for type 2 diabetes (non-insulin dependent diabetes mellitus; NIDDM) in the 1990s. In 1994, the number of patients with type 2 diabetes mellitus worldwide was 100 million, and the estimate for the year 2010 is 216 million. Consequently, type 2 diabetes will be one of the most challenging public health problems, which imposes significant economical impact in the 21st century.

A recent study evaluated the cost-effectiveness (i.e. the effectiveness for 1 unit cost) of exercise as a health promotion activity. The Center for Disease Control (CDC) summarized and reported that the attributable risk percentage of lower physical activity, hypertension, smoking, and hypercholesterol for the incidence of CHD were 34.6%, 28.9%, 25.6%, and 42.7%, respectively. In comparison to other risk factor interventions, the cost-effectiveness analysis demonstrated that a minimum cost can be achieved through exercise intervention as a prevention of CHD.

In this article, we will review the following topics: 1) epidemiological evidence for the preventive effects of physical activity or physical fitness on the incidence of diabetes mellitus, 2) mechanism underlying improved insulin sensitivity, 3) effects of physical training on insulin resistance syndrome, and 4) compliance with health programs for treatment of diabetes mellitus.

2 Epidemilogical Evidence

a) *Relationship between physical activity or physical fitness and incidence of type 2 diabetes mellitus (Table 1 and Table 2)*

Table 1 Relationship between physical activity and incidence of type 2 diabetes mellitus (NIDDM) from prospective cohort study

Research (sex)	Age (n)	Observation periods (yrs.)	Comparative group	RR / OR * (95%CI)	Reference
• Pennsylvania Alumini Heart Study (M)	39-68 (n = 5, 990)	14	more than 500 kcal/wk in leisure-time activity vs less	0.94 (0.90-0.98)	Helmrich et al. (1991)
• Nurse's Health Study (F)	34-59 (n = 87,253)	8	more than 1 vigorous exercise vs less	0.67 (0.6-0.75)	Manson et al. (1991)
• Physician's Health Study (M)	40-84 (n = 21,271)	5	more than 1 vigorous exercise vs less	0.64 (0.52-0.82)	Manson et al. (1992)
• Honolulu Heart Program (M)	45-68 (n = 6,815)	6	upper quintile of PA vs lower 4 quintile of PA	0.49 * (0.34-0.72)	Burchiel et al. (1995)
• British Regional Heart Study (M)	40-59 (n = 7577)	12.8	physically active vs sedentary	0.4 (0.2-0.7)	Perry et al. (1995)
• Osaka Health Study (M)	35-60 (n = 6,013)	10	regular exercise once a week vs less	0.75 (0.62-0.93)	Okada et al. (2000)
• Postmenopausal Study (F)	55-69 (n = 34,257)	12	physically active vs sedentary	0.69 (0.63-0.77)	Folsomet al. (2000)
• Nurse Health Study (F)	40-65 (n = 70,102)	8	the highest level of PA vs the lowest level of PA	0.74 (0.62-0.89)	Hu et al. (1999)

F: female; M: male; PA: physical activity; RR: retative risk; OR: odds ratio; 95%CI: 95 percent confidence interval

Table 2 Relationship between physical fitness and incidence of impaired fasting glucose and type 2 diabetes mellitus (NIDDM) from prospective cohort study

Research (sex)	Age (n)	Observation periods (yrs.)	Comparative group	Physical fitness index	RR / OR * (95%CI)	Reference
Aerobic Center Longitudinal Study (M)	30-79 (n – 8,663)	6	the highest quintile vs the lowest quintile	exercise tolerance metabolic equivalents	0.37* (2.4-5.8)	Wei et al. (1999)
Tokyo Gas Study (F)	19-59 (n = 9,337)	14	low fitness vs high fitness	estimated VO_{2max}	0.53 (0.4-0.71)	Sawada et al. (2000)

M: male; RR: retative risk; OR: odds ratio

There is a lot of epidemiological and experimental evidence concerning the preventive effect of exercise on diabetes, hypertension and dyslipidemia (Bouchard et al. 1988). However, there are only little data supporting the causal effect of exercise and/or diet intervention on atherosclerosis and subsequent coronary heart disease. Unfavorable lifestyles (diet, physical activity, smoking, and alcohol drinking etc.) increase the risk factors (obesity, hypertension, dyslipidemia, and diabetes mellitus), and finally give rise to the diseases such as stroke and ischemic heart disease. On the other hand, cancer is directly effected by unfavorable lifestyles. In Japan, the above mentioned several diseases are recently called lifestyle-related diseases.

Several prospective cohort studies suggested that physical inactivity and lower physical fitness play an important role in the development of insulin resistance and subsequent type 2 diabetes. Using a large sample of a healthy population, several prospective epidemiological studies demonstrated that the relative risk or odds ratio in physically active (Helmrich et al. 1991; Manson et al. 1991, 1992; Burchiel et al. 1995; Perry et al. 1995; Okada et al. 2000; Folsom et al. 2000; Hu et al. 1999), or a high physical fitness (Wei et al. 1999; Sawada et al. 2000) population was lower than that of a physically inactive or low physical fitness population in both men and women.

b) Randomized intervention study for the prevention of type 2 diabetes mellitus or improvement of glucose tolerance (Table 3)

In the large samples of IGT in China, DaQuing IGT and the Diabetes Intervention Study demonstrated that a statistically lower prevalence rate of NIDDM was found in patients participating in exercise therapy (Pan et al. 1997). The same result was also observed in groups of patients participating in a combination program of diet and exercise therapy. Significant improvement of obesity and glucose tolerance was observed in the Diabetes Prevention Study in Finland using men with obesity and IGT (Eriksson et al. 1999). In the Oslo Diet and Exercise Study using obese subjects, insulin resistance improved in diet therapy, and a combination of diet and exercise therapy (Torjesen et al. 1997). However, it did not improve with only exercise therapy.

Table 3 Effects of long-term randomized intervention trial using diet and/or exercise therapy on incidence of type 2 diabetes mellitus (NDDM)

Research (sex)	Age (n)	Observation periods (yrs.)	Comparative group	Incidence		Reference
• Malmo Feasibility Study (M with IGT)	40 (n = 260)	5	D + E vs Control	D + E Control	10.6 %* 28.6 %*	Eriksson et al. (1991)
• Da Quing IGT and NIDDM study (M and F with IGT)	45.0 ± 9.1 (n = 557)	6	Diet (D), Exercise (E), D + , Control	Diet Exercise D + E Control	44 %* 41 %* 46 %* 68 %*	Pan et al. (1997)
• Finnish Diabetes Prevention Study (M and F with IGT and obesity)	40-65 (n = 522)	3.2	D + E vs control	D + E Control	11.0 %* 23.0 %*	Tuomilehto et al. (2001)
• Diabetes Prevention with Program (M and F IGT and obesity)	> 25	2.8	D + E, Metformin vs Placebo	D + E Metformin Placeo	4.8/100 p.y. @ 7.8/100 p.y. @ 11.8/100 p.y. @	Knowler et al. (2002)

M: male, F: female, *: cumulative incidence, @: person-year

3 Mechanism Underlying Improved Insulin Sensitivity

Skeletal muscle is a major site of insulin action, and up to 85% of infused glucose during a euglycemic hyperinsulinemic clamp test is disposed in the muscle tissue (DeFronzo et al. 1981). An experimental study demonstrated that physical training stimulates glucose transporter (GLUT4) translocation, and GLUT4mRNA expression in skeletal muscle (Goodyear and Kahn 1998; Borghouts and Keizer 1999; Ivy et al. 1999). As a result, insulin sensitivity in the whole body is significantly improved.

a) Acute effect of exercise on glucose uptake

The most important factor in the mechanism by which glucose uptake occurs into the muscle by acute exercise is the promotion of GLUT4 translocation from an intracellular pool to the plasma membrane and transverse tubes (T-tubes) by both muscle contraction and insulin. The signal for the increased insulin sensitivity remains unknown, but it may require the glycogen depletion. The depletion of glycogen may be associated with increased insulin sensitivity (Borghouts and Keizer 1999). Recent studies (Goodyear and Kahn 1998; Hayashi et al. 1999) have proven the evidence supporting a new hypothesis that exercise-stimulated glucose transport is mediated and regulated by 5'AMP-activated protein kinase (AMPK) in skeletal muscle (Fig. 1).

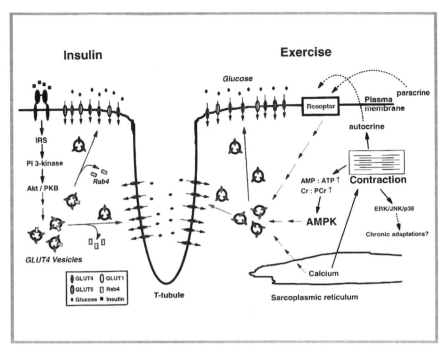

Figure 1. Glucose transporter (GULT4) translocation by insulin and muscle contraction (Goodyear and Kahn 1998; Hayashi et al.1999). Insulin-stimulated GLUT4 translocation involves IRS-1 and PI 3-kinase, and the redistribution of Rab4. Contraction-stimulated GLUT4 translocation does not cause redistribution of Rab4. Recent studies have provided the evidence supporting the new hypothesis that exercise-stimulated glucose transport is mediated and regulated by 5'AMP-activated protein kinase (AMPK).

b) Effect of physical training on insulin sensitivity

Physical training has mostly been shown to improve insulin sensitivity in healthy humans regardless of age, in obese patients, in both insulin dependent diabetes mellitus and NIDDM (Goodyear and Kahn 1998; Borghouts and Keizer 1999). Improvement of insulin sensitivity has generally been considered to be proportional to the rise in physical fitness and VO_2max, and independent of changes in weight and body composition. However, improvement of insulin sensitivity induced by physical training can also be achieved when there are no changes in VO_2max or body mass index. The improvement of insulin sensitivity and glucose tolerance will return to the basal level within a few days after completion of exercise training. However, this can be rapidly regained by one single bout of exercise.

4 Effect of Exercise Training on Insulin Resistance Syndrome (IRS)

a) Effect of exercise training on IRS

Several studies have demonstrated that insulin resistance is a recognized characteristic of several disease states including obesity, type 2 diabetes (NIDDM), essential hypertension, and atherosclerotic cardiovascular disease. Metabolic factors, including hypertension and abdominal distribution of body fat, indicating an elevated risk to develop cardiovascular disease and stroke, are frequently seen in a cluster. This phenomenon is called insulin resistance syndrome (DeFronzo and Ferrannini 1991). Figure 2 shows a schematic summary concerning the contribution of physical activity or fitness on insulin resistance and insulin resistance syndrome, such as diabetes mellitus, dyslipidemia (hypertriglyceridemia and low high-density lipoprotein cholesterol), and hypertension. In addition, a number of other abnormalities, such as hyperuricaemia, microalbuminuria, and hyperfibrinogenaemia, and increased plasminogen activator inhibitor I are also associated with IRS. Several studies have demonstrated beneficial effects of exercise training on IRS (Shahid and Schneider 2000; Eriksson et al. 1997). Exercise-improved insulin sensitivity is also closely linked to the improvement of lipids and lipoprotein metabolism in IGT and type 2 diabetes (Despres and Lamarche 1994).

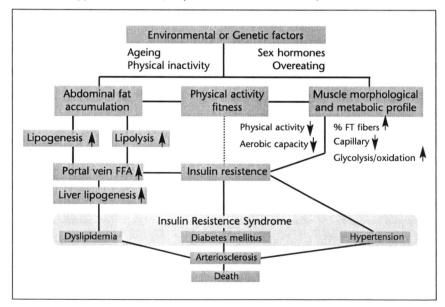

Figure 2. Schematic summary concerning the contribution of physical activity or physical fitness on insulin resistance and insulin resistance syndrome such as

diabetes mellitus, dyslipidemia, hypertension, and other metabolic abnormalities. Physical activities or physical fitness levels is an important contributor for the prevention, development, and improvement of diabetes mellitus through alterations of obesity, especially visceral fat, individual's muscle histochemical and biochemical profiles (such as muscle fiber composition, capillarization, glucose transporter translocation), and glycolytic and oxidative capacity in the muscle. Insulin resistance syndrome is improved by endurance and/or resistance training in both sexes.

b) Role of skeletal muscle profile on insulin resistance

Skeletal muscle has a key role in the consumption of carbohydrates and lipids. Several studies have investigated the relationship between muscle tissue characteristics, and body fat accumulation and/or insulin resistance (Bassett 1994). It has been demonstrated in human and animal experiments that risk factors for the CHD were also significantly associated with fast twitch (FT) muscle fiber, especially FTb fiber (Bassett 1994). In humans, muscle fibers are generally classified as type I (slow twitch; ST) and II (fast-twitch; FT) fibers. The type II fibers are subclassified into type IIA and IIX fibers. Some researchers indicated that the composition of these fiber types is related to the body fat composition and/or insulin-stimulated glucose transport. In fact, the percentage of type I fibers and capillary density is significantly and positively associated with the glucose infusion rate evaluated by hyperinsulinemic eugylycemic clamp (Lillioja et al. 1987).

Type I fibers had higher oxidative potential, and lower glycolytic potential than type II fibers. The GLUT4 content in type I fibers is greater than type II fibers. These results might suggest that muscle fiber composition affected whole body fat oxidation and insulin-stimulated glucose transport. It is considered that the muscle fiber composition is a possible determinant of body fat accumulation and insulin resistance. Mårin et al. (1994) have shown a decreased mitochondrial and capillary density in the skeletal muscle, as well as a decrease in type I to type II fibers in men and women with NIDDM. On the other hand, other studies (Holmäng et al. 1993; Houmard et al 1999) have demonstrated that hyperinsulinemia induces muscle fiber type transformation. It is possible that hyperinsulinemia, which is induced by insulin resistance, alters the muscle fiber types. Further study is needed to elucidate the causal relationship between muscle fiber composition and insulin resistance.

The ratio of glycolytic enzyme activity to oxidative enzyme activity (hexokinase/citrate synthase ratio; HK/CS ratio) is significantly and negatively associated with the glucose infusion rate by clamp method (Simoneau et al. 1995). These ratios (PFK (phosphofructokinase) /CS ratio, and HK /CS ratio etc.) are increased in the order of lean, obese, NIDDM (Simoneau and Kelly 1997) . These results indicate low oxidative enzyme activity is an important factor for the development of insulin resistance.

5 Compliance with Health Program for Treatment of Obesity and Type 2 Diabetes

A combination of diet (low calorie diet and fat restriction etc.) and exercise was the best treatment method for weight and blood glucose control. However, half of the subjects who participated in a program of exercise therapy withdrew from the program during the course of long term treatment. Drop-out rates from the program may even reach 90% after 1 year (Schneider et al. 1992). An epidemiological study has indicated that diabetic patients are less likely to exercise than non-diabetic patients. Recently, it has been emphasized that a psychological approach to weight and blood glucose control programs is beneficial. Key strategies in current behavioral programs on weight reduction and blood glucose control include the following;1) self-monitoring, 2) goal setting, 3) nutrition, 4) exercise, 5) problem solving, 6) cognitive restructuring, and 7) relapse prevention. Eriksson (1999) suggested that the importance of enhancing the levels of routine activities of daily living, such as stair climbing, household chores, and gardening should be emphasized. Some methodological problems of exercise epidemiology and evaluation of health programs are presented in Table 4.

Table 4 Problems of health-related exercise epidemiology and evaluation of health-related exercise program.

1. **Research design in epidemiological study**
   To investigate the direct effect of exercise on the prevention of disease, using randomized control trial methods in population.

2. **Planning of health program**
   Proposing the health program to maintain the exercise habit

3. **Evaluation (economical evaluation) of health program**
   To elucidate the purpose, comparison, and criteria of the evaluation of the health program

6 Conclusion

From this evidence based on epidemiological and experimental studies, it is concluded that exercise, as well as diet therapy contribute to the prevention and improvement of obesity, impaired glucose tolerance (IGT) and type 2 diabetes. Finally, to maintain the continuity of a health program for treatment of obesity and type 2 diabetes, it is necessary to consider the psychological approach to weight and blood glucose control programs.

REFERENCES

Bassett, D.R. (1994). Skeletal muscle characteristics: relationships to cardiovascular risk factors. *Medicine and Science in Sports and Exercise* 26:957-966.

Borghouts, L.B., and Kelzer, H.A. (1999). Exercise and insulin sensitivity: a review. *International Journal of Sports Medicine* 20:1-12.

Bouchard, C., Shepard, R.J., Stephens, T., Sutton, J.R., and McPherson, B.D. Eds. (1988). *Exercise, Fitness, and Health.* Human Kinetics Book, Champaign, Illinois.

Burchiel, C.M., Sharp, D.S., Curb, J.D., Rodriguez, B.L., Hwang, L.J., Marcus, E.B., and Yano, K. (1995). Physical activity and incidence of diabetes: the Honolulu Heart Program. *American Journal of Epidemiology* 141, 360-368.

DeFronzo, R.A., and Ferrannini, E. (1991). Insulin resistance. A multifaceted syndrome responsible for NIDDM, obesity, hypertension, dyslipidemia, and atherosclerotic cardiovascular disease. *Diabetes Care* 14:173-194.

DeFronzo, R.A., Jaqot, E., Jequier, E., Maeder, E., Wahren, J., and Felber, J.P. (1981). The effect of insulin and glucose on the disposal on intravenous glucose. *Diabetes* 30:1000-1007.

Despres, J.-P., and Lamarche, B. (1994). Low-intensity endurance exercise training, plasma lipoproteins and risk of coronary heart disease. *Journal of Internal Medicine* 236:7-22.

Eriksson, K.F., and Lindgarde, F. (1991). Prevention of type 2 (non-insulin-dependent) diabetes mellitus by diet and physical exercise. The 6-year Malmo feasibility study. *Diabetologia* 34:891-8.

Eriksson, J., Taimela, S., and Koivisto, V.A. (1997). Exercise and the metabolic syndrome. *Diabetologia* 40:125-135.

Eriksson, J.G. (1999). Exercise and treatment of type 2 diabetes mellitus; an update. *Sports Medicine* 27:381-391.

Folsom, A.R., Kushi, L.H., and Hong, C-H. (2000). Physical activity and incident diabetes mellitus in postmenopausal women. *American Journal of Public Health* 90:134-138.

Goodyear, L., and Kahn, B.B. *(1998).* Exercise, glucose transport, and insulin sensitivity. Annual Review of Medicine *49:235-261.*

Hayasi, T., Higaki, Y., and Goodyear, R. (1999). Exercise regelation of skeletal muscle glucose transporter. *Advanced in Exercise and Sports Physiology* 5: 1-8.

Helmrich, S.P., Ragland, D.R., Leung, R.W., and Paffenbarger, R.S.Jr. (1991). Physical activity and reduced occurrence of non-insulin-dependent diabetes mellitus. *New England Journal of Medicine* 325:147-152.

Holmang, A., Brzezinska, Z., and Björntorp, P. (1993) Effects of hyperinsulinemia on muscle fiber composition and capillarization in rats. Diabetes, 42:1073-1081.

Houmard, J.A., O'Neiell, D.S., Zheng, D., Hickey, M.S., and Dohm, G.L. (1999). Impact of hyperinsulinemia on myosin heavy chain gene regulation. *Journal of Applied Physiology* 86:1828-1832.

Hu, F.B., Sigal, R.J., Rich-Edwards, J.W, Colditz, G.A., Solomon, C.G., Willett, W.C., Speizer, F.E., and Manson, J.E. (1999). Walking compared with vigorous physical activity and risk of type 2 diabetes in women. *Journal of American Medical Association* 282:1433-1439.

Ivy, J.L., Zderic, T.W., and Fogt, D.L. (1999). Prevention and treatment of non insulin dependent diabetes mellitus. *Exercise and Sports Science Reviews* 27: 1-35.

Knowler, W.C., Barret-Connor, E., Fowler, S.E., Hamman, R.F., Lachin, J.M., Walker, E.A., and Nathan, D.M. (2002). Reduction in the incidence of type 2 diabetes with lifestyle intervention or metformin. *New England Journal of Medicine* 346:393-403.

Lillioja, S., Young, A.A., Gutler, C.L., Ivy, J.L., Abott, W.G.H., Zawadzki, J.K., Yki-Jarvinen, H., Christin, L., Secomb, T.W., and Bogardus, C. (1987). Skeletal muscle capillary density and fiber type are possible determinants of in vivo insulin resistance in man. *Journal of Clinical Investigation* 80:415-424.

Manson, J.E., Rimm, E.B., Stampfer, M.J., Colditz, G.A., Willett, W.C., Kolewski, A.S., Rosner, B., Hennekens, C.H., and Speizer, F.E. (1991). Physical activity and incidence of non-insulin-dependent diabetes mellitus in women. *Lancet* 338:774 -778.

Manson, J.E., Nathan, D.M., Kolewski, A.S., Stampfer, M.J., Willett, W.C., and Hennekens, C.H. (1992). A prospective study of exercise and incidence of diabetes among US male physicians. *Journal of American Medical Association* 268:63-67.

Mårin, P., Andersson, B., Krotkiewski, M., and Björntrop, P. (1994). Muscle fiber composition and capillary density in women and men with NIDDM. *Diabetes Care* 17:382-386.

Okada, K., Hayashi, T., Tsumura, K., Suematsu, C., Endo, G., and Fujii, S. (2000). Leisure-time physical activity at weekends and the risk of type 2 diabetes mellitus in Japanese men: the Osaka Health Survey. *Diabetic Medicine* 17:53-58.

Pan, X. R., Li, G. W., Hu, Y. H., Wang, J. X., Yang, W. Y., An, Z. X., Hu, Z. X., Lin, J., Xiao, J. Z., Cao, H. B., Lui, P. A., Jiang, X. G., Jiang, Y. Y., Wang, J. P., Zheng, H, H., Zhang, H., Bennet, P. H., and Howard, B. V. (1997). Effects of diet and exercise in preventing NIDDM in people with impaired glucose tolerance. The Da Quing IGT and Diabetes Study. *Diabetes Care* 20:537-44.

Perry, I.J., Wannamethee, S.G., Walker, M.K., Thomson, A.G., Whinncup, P.H., and Shaper, A.G. (1995). Prospective study of risk factors for development of non-insulin dependent diabetes in middle aged British men. *British Medical Journal* 310:560-564.

Sawada, S., Muto, T., Tanaka, H., and Blair, S.N. (2000). Cardiorespiratory fitness and incidence of diabetes in Japanese men. *Medicine and Science in Sports and Exercise* 32:S118.

Schneider, S.H., Kachadrurian, A.V., Amorosa, L.F., Clemow, L., and Ruderman, N. B. (1992). Ten-year experience with an exercise-based outpatients life-style modification program in the treatment of diabetes mellitus. *Diabetes Care* 15 (Suppl. 4):1800-1810.

Shahid, S.K., and Schneider, S H. (2000). Effect of exercise on insulin resistance syndrome. *Coronary Artery Disease* 11:103-109.

Simoneau, J.A., Colberg, S.R., Thate, F.L. and Kelly, D.L. (1995). Skeletal muscle glycolytic and oxidative enzyme capacities are determinants of insulin sensitivity and muscle composition in obese women. *FASEB Journal* 9: 273-278.

Simoneau, J.A. and Kelly, D.E. (1997). Altered glycolytic and oxidative capacities of skeletal muscle contribute to insulin resistance in NIDDM. *Journal of Applied Physiology* 83:166-171.

Tuomilehto, J., Lindstrom, J., Eriksson, J.G., Valle, T.T., Hamalainen, H., Ilanne-Parikka, P., Keinanen-Kiukaanniemi, S., Laakso, M., Louheranta, A., Rastas, M., Salminen, V., Uusitupa, M. (2001). Prevention of type 2 diabetes mellitus by changes in lifestyle among subjects with impaired glucose tolerance. *New England Journal of Medicine* 344:1343-50.

Wei, M., Gibbons, L.W., Mitchell, T.L., Kampert, J.B., Lee, C.D., and Blair, S.N. (1999). The association between cardiorespiratory fitness and impaired fasting glucose and type 2 diabetes mellitus in men. *Annals of Internal Medicine* 130:89-96.

Exercise and Cancer

Zsolt Radak[1], Denes Tolvaj[1], Helga Ogonovszky[1], Anna Toldy[1]
AND Albert W. Taylor[2]

[1] Lab. Exercise Physiology, Semmelweis University, Faculty of Physical Education and Sport Science,
[2] Budapest, Hungary,
Dept. Physiology, Faculty of Health Sciences, University of Western Ontario, London, Canada

Correspondence to:

Zsolt Radak, Ph.D.
Lab. Exercise Physiology
Semmelweis University
Faculty of Physical Education and Sport Science Budapest
Hungary
Fax: + + 3613566337
e-mail: radak@mail.hupe.hu

Summary

The development of cancer is dependent upon the combined effects of heredity and environmental factors. However the incidence and the progress of the disease is most probably dependent upon the function of health-promoting genes which maintain the correct production of proteins that sustain the viability of cells and maintain or increase the resistance to damage and damage repair processes. On the other hand, accumulating evidence indicates that environmental factors, lifestyle and especially regular physical exercise can significantly reduce the incidence of cancer, and the extent of prevention or retardation of tumor growth can be as much as 50% for a variety of cancers.

The underlying mechanisms are vague, as to which exercise can reduce the incidence of cancer and/or retard the development of different tumors. Several hypotheses have been proposed and tested, but to date none have proven to be exclusively true and valid. Presently available information would suggest that beneficial effects of exercise on the incidence and development of cancer are mediated through several pathways, including hormonal, immune, energy, and mental systems. It appears that some of the effects might be mediated through redox homeostasis. Exercise likely effects the oncogenes beneficially, but further research is necessary to shed some light on the effects of regular exercise on the incidence of cancer development.

The development of cancer is dependent upon the combined effects of heredity and environmental factors. However the incidence and the progress of the disease, is most probably dependent upon the function of health-promoting genes which maintain the correct production of proteins that sustain the viability of cells and maintain or increase the resistance to damage and damage repair processes.

It has been known in the last 300 years that regular physical exercise decreases the incidence of cancer, due to the appropriate observation of Rammazzini (1700), but even today we do not know much about the exact mechanisms by which exercise mediates the favorable effects. In the last 30 years the number of investigations was significantly increased, however the etiology of cancer partly remains unknown, there a number of uncertainness in the mechanism of natural prevention, treatment and rehabilitation.

On the other hand, accumulating evidence indicate that regular physical exercise can significantly reduce the incidence of cancer, and the extent of prevention or retardation of tumor growth can be as much as 50% percent for a variety of cancers (Shepard and Futzer 1997, Thompson et al. 1995, Radak et al. 2002).

Epidemiological Data on Physical Activity and Cancer

Number of studies has compared the incidence of cancer between physically active and inactive people. The finding of most of the studies revealed that occupational physical activity significantly decreased the incidence of overall cancer risk (Taylor et al. 1962) and this observation was supported by the finding of other studies using variety of occupational physical activity (Wannamethee et al. 1993, Slattery et al. 1988, Steenland et al. 1995, Paffenbarger et al. 1987, Kampert et al. 1996, Blair et al. 1989, Albanes et al. 1989). It has been revealed that an intensity-associated relationship exist between the physical activity and drop in the incidence of over all cancer risk (Slattery et al. 1988). Regular physical occupational or habitual activities effect the incidence of cancer in a site-specific manner. The reduction in incidence of colon cancer can reach as much as 70% for the favor of physically active population and a dose dependent benefit was reported (Arbman et al. 1993, Fraser and Pearce 1993., Lee et al 1991, Peters et al. 1989, Slattery et al. 1988, Vena et al. 1985). Moreover, the long-term physical activity result in greater drop in the incidence of colon cancer than short-term activity (Lee et al. 1991). The incidence of prostate cancer can also reduced by up to 70% by long-term regular physical exercise (Ilic et al. 1996, Le Marchand 1997, Lund Nilsen et al. 2000). The decrease of the incidence of breast cancer goes up to 50% (Carpenter et al. 1999, Berstein et al. 1994, Inger Aeiliv 1997). Epidemiological findings are indicating that regular physical exercise could result in significant decrease in the incidence of lung cancer (Lee et al. 1994, Lee et al. 1999, Severson et al. 1989, Thune and Lund 1997).

Therefore, the available data from epidemiological studies strongly suggests that regular physical activity decreases the incidence of different types of cancer (Table 1) and so far there is no evidence, which proves that regular exercise training result in an increase in cancer incidence.

Szent-Gyorgyi (1968) suggested many years ago that charge transfer (electron transfer) is the reason why cancer cells are unable to arrest growth and commit suicide by apoptosis. Hence, the formation and role of reactive oxygen and nitrogen species (RONS) as an electron acceptors, in the development of cancer appears to be important. The oxidative modifications to macromolecules, or the induction of redox sensitive signaling pathways likely are involved in the development and progress of this uncontrolled proliferation. RONS-induced cellular alterations, especially the oxidative damage of DNA, may underpin certain cancers, and result in the loss of function of tumor suppressor genes and activation of tumor promoting genes with subsequent malignancy (Ames et al. 1993).

Antioxidant therapies presented to cancer-bearing animals have controversial effects (Gerber 2000). Depending on the timing or the type of cancer, antioxidants can promote or retard the development of tumors (Gerber 2000). Regular exercise is known to increase the activity of antioxidant enzymes (Ji and Hollander 2000). Hence, this phenomenon up-regulates the protection against the activity of RONS. Similarly to antioxidant administration, regular exercise could also promote and/or retard the development of certain cancers, depending on the timing and maybe on the intensity of the exercise (Thompson et al. 1995). Therefore, it seems to be appropriate to suggest that physical exercise has beneficial effects, in some part, act trough the RONS, antioxidant and oxidative damage repair systems.

Recently findings from an emerging research area, cellular signaling, has revealed that RONS are necessary for the activation of certain redox proteins, which are obligatory to shift the cells from the resting state to a proliferating state. Moreover, certain genes that are involved in the regulation of apoptosis are also affected by RONS. Gene expression of certain inflammatory agents are also regulated by redox sensitive proteins and the production of inflammatory and anti-inflammatory cytokines could significantly alter the immune system. The effectiveness of the immune system could filter the effects of certain carcinogens and hence the incidence of cancer. Regular exercise is a well known regulator of the immune system. Hence it has been suggested that exercise might decrease the incidence of cancer by the up-regulation of immune system. It seems appropriate to suggest, that regular exercise-induced beneficial effects on cancer development and incidence are not due to one particular pathway, but most probably are the result of several mechanisms which are somehow altered by regular exercise. The etiology of cancer might pinpoint the mechanisms where the exercise-induced alteration can execute modification and alter the development of cancer.

Table 1

Physical activity and incidence of cancer

Pysical activity	Subjects	Results	References
physical activity	212 women	protective againts breast cancer	Kocic, 1996
occupational physical activity	903 women	modest association between intensity of jobs and breast cancer	Coogan, 1999
recreational physical activity	6160 women	reduce risk of breast cancer	Breslow, 2001
recreational exercise	1065 female	no association between breast cancer and exercise	McTieman, 1996
physical activity	25624 women	reduce risk of breast cancer	Thune, 1997
leisure time physical activity	1708 women	not support protective effect againts breast cancer	Chen, 1997
physical activity	25-42 years follow up	not support link between breast cancer and physical activity	Rockhill, 1998
recreational physical activity	3173 women	not support any effet of physical activity on breast cancer	Gammon, 1998
lifetime exercise activity	2027 women	from 17,6 MET/hours activity reduce risk of breast cancer	Carpenter, 1999
physical activity	females aged 50-74	modest association with prevalence of colorectal adenomas	Enger, 1997
physical activity	4246 women	reduce risk of MSI colon cancer	Slattery, 2001
physical activity	326 patients	reduce risk of colon cancer	Tang, 1999
physical activity	1225 patient	protective againts colon cancer	Tavani, 1999
leisure time physical activity	4077 women	reduce risk of endometrial cancer	Moradi, 2000
physical activity	13905 male	lower risk of lung cancer	Lee, 2001
frequency of exercise (sweat)	22071 men	increased physical activity reduce risk of prostate cancer	Liu, 2000
physical activity	5377 men	inactivity elevate risk of prostate cancer	Clarke, 2001
physical activity	20-80 years old men	physical activity protects againts prostate cancer	Oliveria, 1996
physical activity	29133 men	protective effet againts prostate cancer	Hartman, 1998
physical activity	47542 men	no influence on prostate cancer	Giovannucci, 1998
physical activity	709 participants	physical act. has no effect on prostate cancer, not protective	Lacey, 2001

The Etiology of Cancer

Tumors can be divided into three groups according to their biological behavior (Kumar-Cotran-Robbins, 1992). In the first stage, benign, the cells are unable to properly arrest growth resulting in an expanded focus of abnormal cells. Due to the failure of apoptosis immortalization takes place (Hayflick and Moorhead, 1965) causing the development of certain tumors, such as ovarian cysts, and melanocytic nevus (mole) (Swerdlow and Green, 1987).

In the second stage, intermediate, the balance is further disrupted in the cell causing unlimited proliferation and unregulated growth. The surrounding tissues are still not affected, and they represent an ability to digest basement membranes by their enzymatic systems (Tierney, McPhee, Papadakis et al. 1996). Tumors from this stage, for example basal cell carcinoma - the most common type of the non-benign skin tumors (Fleming et al, 1994) can be relatively well controlled by therapeutic agents.

In the third stage, the malignant stage, proliferation is unlimited and this is accompanied by immortalized cell lines. However, in this stage there is acquisition of the mobility to reach and penetrate blood vessel walls for dispersal by the haematogenous and/or lymphogenous systems resulting in malignancy (Fidler, 1990).

Disregarding the conditions above, cancer is a disorder of regulation of cell division and differentiation. Inexorable cell multiplication provides the cell populations by which secondary characteristics appear that enable the evolving neoplasm to exploit a growing disregard for tissue and cellular restraints. By invasion and spread it leads to serious damage and often death of the organism. The main distinctive feature of malignant tumors versus benign tumors is the metastasizing ability.

Genetic Changes

Although proliferation is a basic behavior of cells in nature, most human cells like neurons, adult heart muscle cells, and cells in the upper part of the skin. are unable to proliferate. Under normal conditions only some types of cells have the ability to proliferate. For example epithelial cells in the colon, basal cells of the skin, and stem cells in the bone marrow (Kumar-Cotran-Robbins, 1992). How is it possible that this well-regulated strictly controlled mechanism of proliferation could go wrong and a single cell could change to form an expanding mass of tumor cells, which destroy the whole organism? Loeb et al (1974) have proposed that in the beginning of the tumor progression there is an expression of a mutator phenotype, which causes mutations in genes that normally function in regulating and stabilizing genetic integrity. The integrity of DNA can be altered in normal cells and this might generate mutator phenotypes, which include DNA damage due to inproper DNA synthesis and/or inadequate repair. Errors in DNA synthesis are the result of misincorporation of nucleotides by DNA polymerases. If these errors are not repaired, mutations occur. Very significant amount of DNA damage occur in normal cells due to the interaction of DNA and RONS and a certain amount of oxidative DNA damage has mutagenic potential (Ames et al. 1993, Radak et al. 2001).

In normal cells the rate of mutation is low. However, a significant number of mutations are detected in various cancers (Loeb 1999). Therefore, it appears that cancer cells exhibit mutator phenotype, which leads to the genetic evolution of cancer cells and progress of the tumors (Loeb 1999).

Cancer is a complex disease, which is probably the result of a number of alterations of varying magnitude. The homeostatic balance of oncogenes, tumor suppressor genes, and telomerase is important in the cancer process.

Oncogenes

Genes are able to generate tumor development. For each oncogene there is a normal cellular counterpart, termed proto-oncogene, which functions in normal proliferation, or in many cases, only during the developmental stages (for instance in the uterus) of the organism. It should be noted, that the name may mislead, because the protooncogenes have no being potential hazard, and play an important and vital role in the healing, growth and other homeostatic processes. Normally, cell multiplication requires an exogenous supply of growth factor. The "growth factor" in this text is used in a broad sense, to anabolic hormones such as insulin, steroids and also for transforming growth factor or epidermal transforming factor. To accomplish their effects on a cell, growth factors bind to cell surface receptors. By activating the receptor they initiate a cascade of biochemical events, which leads to DNA synthesis and finally mitosis. (Kumar-Cotran-Robbins , 1992). The epidermal growth factor, for instance, turns on the tyrosine kinase activity of its own receptor. This tyrosine kinase phosphorylates certain tyrosine residues in many transmembrane or cytoplasmatic proteins such as the cytoskeletal protein, vinculin. These phosphorylated proteins act as signal transducers and influence some proteins in the nuclei called transcription factors, which induce, as a last step, DNA synthesis and mitosis. There are examples for proto-oncogen – oncogen transformation on all four levels (Kumar-Cotran-Robbins, 1992), (See Table 2). If the name of the proto-oncogen is, for example, sis, the name of the oncogen is c-sis (cellular oncogen).

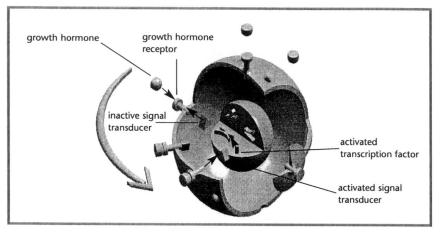

growth hormone

growth hormone receptor

inactive signal transducer

activated transcription factor

activated signal transducer

Figure 1. *The effect of growth hormone on cell.*

Table 2
Oncogenes and cancer

Category	Name of oncogene	Name of onco-protein	Tumor
Growth factor	c-sis	PDGF-b chain	osteosarcoma
Growth factor receptor	c-neu	EGF-like receptor	breast cancer
Signal transducer	c-ras	GTP-binding protein family	colon cancer
Transcription factor	c-myc	not clear	Burkitt-lymphoma

There are a number of mechanisms by which oncogenes could act (Hunter 1991). The cell could produce an abnormal mass of growth factor, and stimulate itself (autocrin stimulation) or the cells around it (paracrin stimulation). For instance: in some type of osteosarcomas, the malignant cells produce Platelet-Derived Growth Hormon b-chain (PDGF) to aid the proliferation. (Kumar-Cotran-Robbins, 1992). The cell can overexpress the growth factor receptors, to misuse the growth hormones circulating in the blood, for example, overexpressed endothelium growth factor-like (EGF) receptor (c-neu) causing breast cancer, ovarian tumors or stomach cancer (Kumar-Cotran-Robbins 1992). The cell can produce mutant signal transducer proteins, to gain independence of different stimuli. One of the most frequent representatives of this method is the c-ras oncogen family, which codes for a family of GTP-binding cell membrane proteins (for example protein p21). This protein is active when binding GTP, but hydrolyzes the bound GTP to GDP to return to the inactive form. An adequate mutation in the proper subunit can enable the hydrolyzing activity of the ras-protein, and the enzyme remains in an excited state, continuously activating the adenilat-cyclase and indirectly stimulating the transcription factors in the nucleus (Taparowsky et al., 1982). It is estimated that for about 50% of colon cancer cases one of these mutant genes is present (Barbacid, 1990). The cell can produce modified transcription proteins for uncontrolled continuous proliferation. For instance, the product of the c-myc oncogene (a transcription factor) can lead to Burkitt-lymphoma (Magrath, 1990).

Tumor suppressor genes

This class of genes is heterogeneous and has only one common feature, which distinguishes them from the proto-oncogenes. Genetic loss of these genes is enough to lead to malignant transformation, and there is no need for an active faulty contribution to cancer development (Marshall 1991). The existing but mutant gene, coding for inactive protein, is also enough to turn on malignancy. Therefore, these genes act a built-in brakes, and without them cell proliferation would occur at an uncontrollable rate. See Table 3 (adopted from Yeo, 1999).

Table 3
Tumor suppressor genes and cancer

Gene	Cancer syndrome	Principal tumors
Rb1	Retinoblastoma	retinoblastoma, osteosarcoma, small cell lung cancer (SCLC).
P53	Li-Fraumeni syndrome	sarcomas, lung cancer, breast and brain tumors
WT-1	Wilms' tumor	Nephroblastoma
BRCA-1	Familial breast cancer	breast and ovarian cancer
BRCA-2	Familial breast cancer	breast (and other ?) cancer

The two most examined and known tumor suppressor genes are the Rb-1 and the p53.

Rb-1

Rb-1 (retinoblastoma gene) is found on the 14th region of the short arm of the 13th chromosome (13q14). Its product pRB (protein Rb) is a DNA-binding protein, which normally inhibits cells for doubling chromosomes, as the first step in mitosis, thus blocking division. The mutant form is inactive and enables the retinal cells to proliferate without stopping. This failure of the Rb-1 gene is responsible for both forms of human retinoblastoma: the familial form (40% of the cases) and for sporadic form 60% (Draper et al., 1986; Friend et al., 1987)). In the sporadic form, the inherited alleles are +/+ (both alleles are normal).

In this two somatic mutations for malignancy, and the onset of the retinoblastoma is in adulthood and the appearance of cancer are dominantly limited on one eye.

In the familial form, the inherited alleles are −/+ (one of the alleles is defective). Only one somatic mutation is needed to bring about malignancy, and the onset of the retinoblastoma is early in life and the cancer damages both eyes often leading to blindness.

It can be concluded that the malignant transformation demands two mutations (two-hit theory: Knudson,1974), but one of these could be inherited. To date there is no case described with two inherited failure alleles: −/−, maybe this genetic constellation causes death in fetal life.

p53

The p53 tumor suppressor gene appears more frequently in human cancer than any other known gene. Approximately 50% of all human tumors carry a p53 mutation and at least 52 different types of tumors have p53mutations (Nigro et al., 1989, Kiellstein at al., 1991, Greenblatt et al., 1994). Many different functions have been attributed to the tumor suppressor gene product, p53, including DNA repair cofactor and exonuclease. But, by far the most significant function attributed to p53 is its role as a transcriptional regulator. p53 is expressed at basal levels in several tissues but in response to stress (for instance: ionizing radiation, chemical agents), p53 levels are induced (MacCallum et al.,1996). Cells respond to p53 induction by undergoing either growth arrest or apoptosis. The choice between growth arrest and apoptosis is thought to be determined, in part by the levels of p53, the proliferation state, and the growth factor environment of the cell (Midgley et al. 1995). In other words, the p53 gene is guarding over the health of the "new-born" cell, and kills its own cell if it necessary (Rodin and Rodin, 2000). The proteins coded by the p53 gene have a DNA-binding subunit, and four proteins form a tetramer unit. If only one of these proteins is faulty, the tetramer is unable to bind to the DNA, and loses its activity. This structural feature leads to an interesting and for a long time unexplainable observation: In tissue cultures, after administration of normal p53 protein, tumor cells lose the ability to proliferate. But, in tissue cultures of benign cells, the administration of mutant p53 protein leads often to malignant transformation of the cells, obviously through the blocking of the activity of the normal p53 proteins (Martinez, 1991).

Telomerase

Whereas normal human somatic cells have a limited proliferative capacity and undergo senescence after a finite number of doublings, most malignant cells show an infinite life-span (Trentin et al. 1999). Replicative senescence is dependent upon cumulative cell division, indicating that proliferation is limited by a "mitotic clock" (Hayflick and Moorhead, 1965; Hayflick, 1997). A key mechanism that controls human somatic cell cycle arrest and limits the life-span of these cells is the progressive shortening of chromosomes at every division, which is due to the inability of DNA polymerase to replicate the 3' ends of linear DNA molecules completely (Greider and Blackburn, 1985; Nugent and Lundbland, 1988). Each cell division results in a loss of 50-200 bp (base pair) of telomere. The name "telomere" means the very end of the chromosomes, and it owns a specialized structure. The telomeres consist of highly conserved tandemly repeated guanosin-rich sequences, in human TTAGGG hexanucleotids (Moyzis et al., 1988). The total size of the telomere is 5 to 15 kbp (kilo base pair) per chromosome end – it means approximately 1000-2500 copies of this hexamer, being associated with specific proteins. The length of the repeated region is highly variable among the chromosomes of single cells and among different cells of a population. (Landsorp et al. 1996). Telomeres are essential for chromosome stability by protecting chromosome ends from the attack of nucleotic enzymes and prevent chromosomes from fusing together (Blackburn, 1991). In normal human somatic cells, increasing cell divisions leads to a decreasing length of telomeres due to incomplete replication of the telomeric ends. In such cells senescence is induced in vitro at a critical minimum telomeric size (Harley, 1991; Allsopp and Harley, 1995). Telomerase, a ribonucleoprotein enzyme, can compensate for the telomere loss by adding new telomeric repeats to the chromosome ends. Cells with unlimited proliferation capacity – the germ-line cells (Chiara et al. 1999), and a large number of human tumors – have been shown to contain active telomerase, whereas in normal human tissues telomeres are short, and telomerase activity is low or undetectable. However, studies indicate that telomerase activity is also detected in normal human somatic cells, such as hematopoietic stem cells (Hiyama et al., 1995; Chiu et al., 1996; Morrison et al., 1996), lymphocytes (Broccoli et al., 1995; Weng et al., 1996; Norrback et al., 1996) and skin epithelial cells (Yasumoto et al.1996; Harle-Bachor and Boukamp; Taylor et al.; 1996), that have self-renewal capability. It seems that there are a few exceptions to this rule, telomere length maintenance needs telomerase as an example have been found, that show permanent cell lines without telomerase activity, thus indicating the possibility of an alternative mechanism for telomere length maintenance. (Kim et al., 1994; Whitaker et al., 1995; Bryan et al. 1995).

Therefore, it is suggested that, in most cases, telomerase is necessary for unlimited division of tumor cells. Normal human tissues do not contain active telomerase and this is why genetic cell mutation is needed for tumor proliferation. Some types of human cells do contain telomerase under normal conditions. In this case tumor development may not demand or de novo syntheses of telomerase, although the exact regulation of this enzyme is still unknown.

Mechanism by which Physical Exercise Affects Cancer

The effects of regular exercise to decrease cancer incidence are well documented. However the underlining mechanisms are vague. Several hypotheses have been proposed and tested, but to date none have proven to be exclusively true and valid. Table 4 contain the results obtained from animal studies, which examined the effects of exercise on different types of cancer. Presently available information, would suggest that beneficial effects of exercise on the incidence and development of cancer is mediated through several pathways.

Table 4
The effects of exercise on variety of cancer in animal model

Physical activity	Animals	Results	References
4-10 week training	<11 male mice	no effect on intestinal polyps	Colbert,2000
60 min training 5 times/week	21-50days old rats	no exercise induced changes in mammary gland development	Whittal,1996
8 weeks of 2 km/day running	8 week old rats	Risk of neoplasm and carcinoma reduced	Thorling,1994
physical exercise	5 week old rats	reduce hepatocarcinogenesis	Sugie,1992
wheel exercise	female rats	Had no effect on overall tumor incidence	Cohen,1993
8 months running wheel exercise	5 week old rats	preventive effect on oxygen toxicity	Suzuki,1992
5 times a week progressive running exercise	21-50 days old rats	no effect on tumor burden but on tumor growth rate	Whittal,1998
3 month 5 times a week treadmill exercise	female rats	cancer incidence reduced by 35%,multiplicity by<60%	Thompson,1995
4 months running wheel exercise	28 days old rats	exercise had little effect on pancreatic tumorigenesis than diet	Giles,1992
3 times a week exercise for 7 weeks	tumor bearing rats	May have initial protection in retarding tumor growth	Deuster,1985
wheel activity	rats	reduced colon cancer risk	Andrianopoulus, 1987
wheel exercise for 4 months	male and female rats	voluntary exerc. reduced the growth rate of pancreatic foci	Roebuck,1990
38 week of wheel exercise	5 week old rats	incidence of colon carcinogenesis and liver foci were inhibited	Reddy,1988
running exercise	no information	prevent ethanol induced increased risk for hepatic cancer	Duncan,1997

Aerobic physical exercise decreases the level of circulating testosterone which has been implicated in prostate cancer. Administration of anabolic steroids, therefore, imposes a threat of increased incidence of prostate cancer. Therefore, it could be suggested that aerobic exercise, exercise of low intensity and long duration, might be effective by decreasing the effects of testosterone on prostate cancer, which seems to be well documented (Gann et al. 1996, Le Marchand et al. 1991).

Other sex hormones like progresterone and estradiol are implicated in the etiology of breast cancer. Regular exercise appears to be very effective in decreasing the incidence of breast cancer and the regulatory role of exercise might mediate this beneficial effect.

Regular exercise induces favorable effects on insulin, and prostaglandin and hence can effect growth and proliferation of colonic cells and thus decrease the incidence of colon cancer. Moreover, exercise might stimulate gastric movement and then decrease the time of fecal mass in the colonic regions, and thus be important in decreasing the incidence of colon cancer.

There are only a few reports, which have examined the effects of exercise on oncogenes. Leukemic solid tumor-bearing mice were assigned to control, exercise trained and continuously exercising group. The size of the tumors of the continuously exercising group was 50% smaller than that of the control mice. The Ras content of the smaller tumor was significantly higher than in the larger tumors of the control animals (Radak et al. 2000). Therefore, it appears that exercise training modulates the oncogene proteins in tumors and by this retards the development of the tumors. In concert to Ras the content of I-kappa B also was higher in tumors of continuously exercising mice. Hence, it is suggested that redox sensitive transcription is also modulated by physical exercise and this contributes to the tumor growth-retarding effects of exercise. Aging appears to increase the DNA binding of the nuclear transcription factor kappa B in skeletal muscle and liver of rats. Regular exercise attenuates this age-associated increase in liver but not in skeletal muscle (Radak et al. unpublished observation) indicating that exercise effects the transcription of certain genes.

The content of p53 is relatively small in cells, so it is difficulty to reliably measure. On the other hand, the mutant form of p53 has a significantly longer half-life and it tends to accumulate in cells. The mutant form of p53 is not significantly altered in tumors of leukemic mice or in liver of leukemic sarcoma tumor-bearing mice (Radak et al. 2001).

Telomerase activity, which often increased in cancer cells is not altered in liver of exercising, or sarcoma solid tumor-bearing animals (Radak et al. 2001). We exposed rats to severe exercise training but the activity of telomerase was not changed, indicating that physical exercise does not induce a stress, to alter telomerase activity.

The activity of antioxidant enzymes in the tumor of leukemia bearing mice was not significantly altered by physical exercise, which suggests that the difference in tumor progression is not accompanied by altered oxidant production suggested from the activity of antioxidant enzymes. On the other hand, the accumulation of oxidative damage of macromolecules, proteins, lipids and DNA, showed some difference in the tumor. The level of lipid peroxidation was low in larger tumors compared with small tumors of exercising animals (Radak et al. 2002). Interestingly, the extent of oxidative protein damage, judged by the accumulation of reactive carbonyl derivatives, showed a opposite trend, namely, the small tumors had lower levels of carbonyls than large tumors. The overall carbonyl concentration was about three fold higher in tumors than in normal tissues. The nuclear DNA damage, measured by 8-hydroxydeoxyguanosine, was not different in the tumors. The data on antioxidant enzymes, and oxidative damage markers, suggest, that in leukemic tumors the formation of RONS might not be significant and the some difference in the oxidative repair process is plausible.

Exercise therefore could alter oncogenes, transcription factors and by this alter the development of certain tumors. Thus, it cannot be ruled out that physical exercise mediates beneficial effects through the alteration of oncogenes, proto-oncognes and transcription factors. It is also possible that exercise-induced alterations in RONS production are involved in the progression of the disease.

Summary

The available epidemiological and direct experimental data suggest that regular exercise has the capability to significantly decrease the incidence of certain cancers. Despite intensive investigation, the mechanism(s) remain vague. It is suggested that, exercise probably acts through many different pathways, including hormonal, immune, energy, and mental systems. It appears that some of the effects might be mediated by the effects of exercise on the rate of RONS production, antioxidant and oxidative damage repair systems, including DNA repair. Exercise likely effects the oncogenes beneficially. However the involvement of exercise-induced control in telomerase activity appears unlikely. Unquestionably, further research is necessary to shed some light on the effects of regular exercise on the incidence of cancer development.

REFERENCES

Albanes, D., Blair, A., and Taylor, P. R. (1989). Physical activity and risk of cancer in the NHANES 1 population. *American Journal of Public Helath*, Vol., 79., pp. 744-750.

Allsopp, R C and Harley, C. B. (1995). Evidence of a critical telomere length in senescent human fibroblasts. *Experimental Cell Research*, Vol., 219., pp. 130-136.

Ames, B.N., Shinegawa, M:K., and Hagen, T.M. (1993). Oxidants, antioxidants and the degenerative diseases of aging. *Proceedings of the National Academy of Sciences of the USA.* Vol., 90., pp. 7915-7922.

Andrianopoulos G., Nelson, R. L., Bombeck, C. T., Souza, G. (1987). The influence of physical activity in 1,2 dimethylhydrazine-induced colon carcinogenesis in rat. *Anticancer Research Jul-Aug Vol.,7(4B)*, pp. 849-52.

Arbman, G., Axelson, O., Fredriksson, M., Nilsson, E., and Sjodahl, R. (1993). Do occupational factors influence the risk of colon and rectal cancer in different ways? *Cancer* Vol., 72., pp. 2543-2549.

Barbacid, M. (1990). Ras oncogenes: Their role in neoplasia. *European Journal of Clinical Investigation*, Vol., 20., pp. 225-235.

Bernstein, L., Henderson, B. E., Hanisch, R., Sullivan-Halley, J., and Ross, R.K (1994). Physical exercise and reduced risk of breast cancer in young women. *J. Natl Cancer Inst.* Vol.,86., pp. 1403-1408.

Blackburn, E. H. (1991). Structure and function of telomeres. Nature, Vol.,350.,pp. 569-573. Blair. S. N., Kohl, H. W., Paffenbarger, R. S., Clark, D. G., Cooper, K. H., and Gibbons, L. W. (1989): Physical fitness and all-causemortality. A prospective study of healthy men and women. *Journal of Americal Medical Assotiation*, Vol., 262., pp. 2395-2401.

Breslow,R.A., Ballard-Barbash R., Munoz, K., Graubard, B. I. (2001). Long term recreational physical activity and breast cancer in the National Health and Nutrition Examination Survey I. epidemiological follow up study. *Cancer-Epidemiol-Biomarkers-Prev* Jul Vol.,10(7), pp. 805-8.

Broccoli, D., Young, J. W. and de Lange, T. (1995). Telomerase activity in normal and malignant hematopoietic cells. *Proceedings of the National Academy of Sciences of the USA*, Vol. 92., pp. 9082-9086.

Bryan, T. M., Englezou, A., Gupta, J., Bacchetti, S. and Reddel, R. R. (1995). Telomere elongation in immortal human cells without detectable telomerase activity. *EMBO Journal*, Vol. 14., pp. 4240-4248.

Carpeneter, C. L., Ross R. K., Paganini-Hill, A., Bernstein, L. (1999). Lifetime exercise activity and breast cancer risk among post-menopausal women. *British Journal of Cancer* Aug Vol. 80(11), pp. 1852-8.

Carpenter, C. L., Ross, R. K., Paganini-Hill, A., and Bernstein, L. (1999). Lifetime exercise activity and breast cancer risk among post-menopausal women. *British Journal of Cancer* Vol. 80., pp. 1852-1858.

Chen, C. L., White, E., Malone, K. E., Daling, J. R. (1997). Leisure-time physical activity in relation to breast cancer amoung young women (Washington,US). *Cancer Couses Control* Jan Vol. 8(1), pp. 77-84.

Chiara, M., Chariklia, P., Daniela, M., Esftathios, S. G., Claudio, F., and Fiorella, N. (1999). Telomere Length in Fibroblasts and Blood Cells from Healthy Centenarians. *Experimental Cell Research*, Vol. 248., pp. 234-242.

Chiu, C. P., Dragowska, W., Kim, N. W., Vaziri, H., Yui, J., Thomas, E. T., Harley, C. B. and Landsorp, P. M. (1996). Differential expression of telomerase activity in hematopoietic progenitors from adult human bone marrow. *Stem Cells*, Vol. 14., pp. 239-248.

Clarke, G., Whittemore, A.S. (2001). Prostate cancer risk in relation to anthropometry and physical activity the National Health and Nutrition Examination Survey I. epidemiological follow up study. *Cancer-Epidemiol-Biomarkers*-Prev Sep Vol. 9(9), pp. 875-81.

Cohen L. A. et al. (1993). Inhibition of rat mammary tumorgenesis by voluntary exercise. *In Vivo* Mar-Apr Vol. 7(2), pp.151-8.

Colbert, L. H., Davis, J. M., Essig, D. A., Ghaffar, A., Mayer, E. P. (2000). Exercise and tumor development in a mouse predisposed to multiple intestinal adenomas.. *Medicine and Science in Sports and Exercise* Oct Vol., 32 (1), pp. 1704-8.

Coogan, P. F., Aschengran, A. (1999). Occupational physical activity and breast cancer risk in Upper Cape Cod cancer incidence study. *Americal Journal of International Medicine* Aug Vol. 36(2), pp. 279-85.

Deuster P.A., Morison S.D., Ahrens R.A. (1985). Endurance exercise modifies cachexia of tumor growth in rats. *Medicine and Science in Sports and Exercise* Jun Vol. 17(3), pp. 385-92.

Draper, G. J., Sanders, B. M. and Kingsdom, J. E. (1986). Second primary neoplasms in patients with retinoblastoma. *British Journal of Cancer*, Vol. 53., pp. 661-671.

Duncan, K., Harris, S., Ardies, C. M. (1997). Running exercise may reduce risk of lung and liver cancer by inducing activity of antioxidant and phase II. enzymes. *Cancer Letters* Jun24 Vol. 116(2), pp.151-8.

Enger, S. M., Longnecker, M. P., Lee, E. R., Frankl, H. D., Hailer, R. W. (1997). Recent and past physical activity and prevalence of colorectal adenomas. *British Journal of Cancer* Vol. 75(5), pp. 740-5.

Fidler, J. (1990). Critical factors in the biology of human cancer metastasis: Twenty-eighth G.H.A. Clowes Memorial Award Lecture. *Cancer Research*, Vol. 50/19, pp. 6130-6138.

Fleming, D., Amonette, R., Monaghan, T. and Fleming, M. D. (1994). Principles of management of basal and squamous cell carcinoma of the skin. *Cancer*, Vol. 75(2 suppl.), pp. 699-704.

Fraser, G., and Pearce, N. (1993). Occupational physical activity and risk of cancer of the colon and rectum in New Zealand males. *Cancer Causes Control*, Vol. 4., pp. 45-50.

Friend, S. H., Horowitz, J. M., Gerber, M. R., Wang, X. F., Bogenmann, E., Li, F. P. and Weinberg, R. A. (1987). Deletions of a DNA sequence in retinoblastomas and mesenchymal tumors: Organization of the sequence and its encoded protein. *Proceedings of the National Academy of Sciences of the USA*, Vol. 84., pp. 9059-9063.

Gammon, M. D., John, E. M., Britton, J. A. et al (1998). Recreational physical activity and breast cancer risk among women under 45 years. *American Journal of Epidemiology* Feb1 Vol. 147(3), pp. 273-80.

Gann PH, Hennekens CH, Ma J, Longcope C, Stampfer MJ. (1996). Prospective study of sex hormone levels and risk of prostate cancer. J Natl Cancer Inst 88:1118-26

Gerber M. (2000). Oxidative stress, antioxidants and cancer. In: Sen CK, Packer L, Hanninen O eds. *Handbook of Oxidants and Antioxidants in Exercise*. Amsterdam, Elsevier Sci; pp. 927-949.

Giles T.C., Roebuck B.D. (1992). Effect of voluntary exercise and/or food restriction on pancreatic tumorigenesis in male rats. *Advances in Experimental Med-Biol*, Vol. 322., pp.17-27.

Giovannucci, E. Leitzman, M., Spigelman D., Rimm, E. B., Colditz, G. A., Stampfer, M. J., Willett, W. C. (1998). A prospective study of physical activity and prostate cancer in male health professionals. *Cancer Research* Nov15 Vol. 58(22), pp. 5117-22.

Greenblatt, M. S., Bennett, W. P., Hollstein, M. and Harris, C. C. (1994). Mutatios in the p53 tumor suppressor gene: clues to cancer etiology and molecular pathogenesis. *Cancer Research*, Vol. 54., pp. 4855-4878.

Greider, C. W. and Blackburn, E. H. (1985). Identification of a specific terminal transferase activity in Tetrahymena extracts. *Cell*, Vol. 43., pp. 405-413.

Harle-Bachor, C. and Boukamp, P. (1996). Telomerase activity in the regenerative basal layer of the epidermis in human skin and in immortal and carcinoma-derived skin keratinocytes. *Proceedings of the National Academy of Sciences of the USA*, Vol. 93., pp. 6476-6481.

Harley, C. B. (1991). Telomere loss: Mitotic clock or genetic time bomb? *Mutation Research*, Vol. 256., pp. 271-282.

Hartman, T. J., Albanes, D., Rautalahti, M., Tangrea, J. A., Virtamo, J., Stolzenberg R., Taylor, R. R. (1998). Physical activity and prostate cancer in the Alfa-Thocopherol, Beta-Carotine Study (Finland). *Cancer Couses Control* Jan Vol., 9(1),pp.11-8.

Hayflick, L. (1997). Mortality and immortality at the cellular level. A review. *Biochemistry Moscow,*Vol. 62, pp. 1180-1190.

Hayflick, L. and Moorhead, P. S. (1965): The serial cultivation of human diploid cell strains. *Experimental Cell Research*, Vol. 25, pp. 585-621.

Hiyama, K., Hirami, Y., Kyoizumi, S., Akiyama, M., Hiyama, E., Piatyszek, M. A., Shay, J.W., Ishioka, S. and Yamakido, M. (1995). Activation of Telomerase in Human Lymphocytes and Hematopoietic Progenitor Cells. *Journal of Immunology*, Vol. 155, pp. 3711-3715.

Hunter, T. (1991). Cooperation beetween oncogenes. *Cell*, Vol. 64., pp. 249-270.

Ikuyama T., Watanabe, T., Minedishi, Y., Osanai, H. (1993). Effect of voluntary exercise on 3'-methyl-4-dimethylaminoazobenzene-induced hepatomas in male Jc1:Wistar rats. *Proceedings of the Society Experimental Biology and Medicine* Nov Vol. 204(2),pp. 211-5.

Ilic, M., Vlajinac, H., and Marinkovic, J. (1996). Case-control study of risk factors for prostata cancer. *British Journal of Cancer*, Vol. 74., pp.1682-1686.

Inger T. and Eiliv L. Exercise and breast cancer. *New Engl. J. Med.* 1997; 337:708-709.

Ji L.L. and Hollander J. Antioxidant enzyme defense: effects of aging and exercise. In: Radak Z., eds. *Free Radicals in Exercise and Aging.* Champaign, IL. Human Kinetics; 2000:35-72.

Kampert, J. B., Blair, S. N., Barlow, C. E., and Kohl, H. W. (1996). Physical activity, physical fitness and all-cause and cancer mortality: a prospective study of men and women. *Annals of Epidemiology*, Vol. 6., pp. 452-457.

Kiellstein, M., Sidransky, D., Vogelstein, B. and Harris, C. C. (1991): p53 mutations in human cancers. *Science*, Vol. 253., pp. 49-53.

Kim, N. W., Piatyszek, M. A., Prowse, K. R., Harley, C. B., West, M. D., Ho, P. L. C., Coviello, G. M., Wright, W. E., Weinrich, S. L. and Shay, J. W. (1994). Specific association of human telomerase activity with immortal cells and cancer. *Science*, Vol. 266., pp. 2011-2015.

Knudson, A.G. Jr. (1974). Heredity and human cancer. *American Journal of Pathology*, Vol. 77(1)., pp. 77-84.

Kocic, B, Jankovic, S., Petrovic, B., Tiodorovic, B., Filipovic, S. (1996). The significance of physical activity and anthropomertic parameters for the development of breast cancer. *Vojnosanit-Pregl.* Jul-Aug Vol. 53(4), pp. 301-4.

Kumar-Cotran-Robbins (1992): Basic Pathology. W. B. Saunders Company, Philadelphia, Pennsylvania, USA

Lacey, J. V., Dedng, J., Dosemeci, M., Gao, Y. T., Mostofi, F. K., Sesterhenn, I. A., Xie, T., Hsing, A. W. (2001). Prostate cancer, benign prostatic hyperplasia and physical activity in Shanghai, China. *International Journal of Epidemiology* Apr Vol. 30(2), pp. 341-9.

Landsorp, P. P. M., Verwoerd, N. P., van de Rijke, F. M., Dragowska, W., Little, M. T., Dirks, R. W., Raap, A. K. and Tanke, H. J. (1996). Heterogeniety in telomere length of human chromosomes. *Human Molecular Genetics*, Vol. 5. pp. 685-691.

Le Marchand, L., Kolonel, L. N., and Yoshizawa, C. K. (1991). Lifetime occupational physical activity and prostate cancer risk. *American Journal of Epidemiology,* Vol. 133., pp. 103-111.

Lee, I. M., R. S. Paffenberger R.S. Jr, and Hsieh C. (1991). Physical activity and risk of developing colorectal cancer among college alumni. *J. Natl. Cancer Inst.*, Vol. 83., pp. 1324-1329.

Lee, I. M., Paffenbarger RS Jr. (1994). Physical activity and its relation to cancer risk: a prospective study of college alumni. Medicine Science in Sport and Exercise 26:831-837.

Lee, I. M., sesso H.D., Paaffenberger RS, Jr. (2001). Physical activity and risk of lung cancer. *International Journal of Epidemiology* Jan1 Vol. 31(1), pp. 126-30.

Liu, S., Lee, I. M., Linson, P., Ajani, u., Buring, J. E., Hennekens, C. H. (2000). A prospective study of physical activity and risk of prostate cancer in US physicians *International Journal of Epidemiology* Feb Vol. 29(1), pp. 29-35.

Loeb, L. A. (1991). Mutator phenotype may be reguired for multistage carcinogenesis. *Cancer Research*, Vol. 51., pp. 3075-3079.

Loeb, L. A., Springgate, C.F., and Battula, N. (1974). Errors in the DNA replication as a basis of a malignant change. *Cancer Research*, Vol. 34., pp. 2311-2321.

Lund Nilsen, T. I., Johnsen, R., and Watten, L. J. (2000). Socio-economic and lifestyle factors associated with the risk of prostate cancer. *British Journal of Cancer*, Vol. 82., pp. 1358-1363.

MacCallum, D. E., Hupp, T.R., Midgley, C. A., Stuart, D., Campbell, S. J., Harper, A., Walsh, F. S., Wright, E. G., Balmain, A., Lane, D. P. and Hall, P. A. (1996). The p53 response to ionising radiation in adult and developing murine tissues. *Oncogene*, Vol. 13., pp. 2575-2587.

Magrath (1990). The pathogenesis of Burkitt's lymphoma. *Advances in Cancer Research*, Vol. 55., pp. 133-270.

Marshall, C. J. (1991). Tumor suppressor genes. *Cell*, Vol. 64., pp. 313-326.

Martinez, J., Georgoff, I., Martinez, J. and Levine, A. J. (1991). Cellular localization and cell cycle regulation by a temperature-sensitive p53 protein. *Genes and Development.*, Vol. 5., pp. 151-159.

McTieman, A., Stanford, J. L., Weiss, N. S., Daling, J. R., Voigt, L. F.(1996). Occurance of breast cancer in relation to recreational exercise in women age 50-64 years. *Epidemiology* Nov Vol. 7(6), pp. 598-604.

Midgley, C. A., Owens, B., Briscoe, C.V., Thomas, D. B., Lane, D. P. and Hall, P. A. (1995). Coupling between gamma irradiation, p53 induction and the apoptotic response depends upon cell type in vivo. *Journal of Cell Science*, Vol. 108., pp. 1843-1848.

Moradi, T., Weiderpass, E., Signorello, L. B., Persson, I., Nyren, O., Adami, H. O. (2000). Physical activity and promenopausal endometrial cancer risk (Sweden). *Cancer Causes Control* Oct Vol. 11(9), pp. 829-37.

Morrison, S. J., Prowse, K. R., Ho, P. and Weissman, I. L. (1996). Telomerase activity in hematopoietic cells is associated with self-renewal potential. *Immunity*, Vol. 5., pp. 207-216.

Moyzis, R.K., Buckingham, J. M., Cram, L. S., Dani, M., Deaven, L. L., Jones, M. D., Meyne, J., Ratliff, R.-L. and Wu, J. R. (1988). A highly conserved repetitive DNA sequence, TTAGGG)n, present at the telomeres of human chromosomes. *Proceedings of National Academy Science USA.*, Vol. 85., pp. 6622-6628.

Nigro, J. M., Baker, S. J., Preisinger, A. C. et al. (1989). Mutations in the p53 gene occur in diverse human tumour types. *Nature*, Vol. 342., pp. 705-708.

Norrback, K. F., Dahlenborg, K., Carlsson, R. and Roos, G. (1996). Telomerase activation in normal B lymphocytes and non-Hodgkin's lymphomas. *Blood*, Vol. 88., pp. 222-229.

Nugent, C. L. and Lundbland, V. (1988). The telomerase reverse transcriptase; Components and regulation. *Genes and Development*, Vol. 12. pp. 1073-1085.

Oliveria, S. A., Kohl, H. W. 3rd, Trichopoulos, D., Balir, S. N. (1996). The association between cardiorespiratory fitness and prostate cancer. *Medicine and Science in Sports and Exercise* Jan Vol. 28(1), pp. 97-104.

Paffenberger, R. S., JR., Hyde, R. T., and Wing, A. L. (1987). Physical activity and incidence of cancer in diverse populations: a preliminary report. *American Journal of Clinical Nutrition*, Vol. 45., pp. 312-317.

Peters, R. K., Garabrant, D. H., Yu, M. C., and Mack, T. I. V. I. (1989). A case-control study of occupational and dietary factors in colorectal cancer in young men by subsite. *Cancer Researche*, Vol. 49., pp. 5459-5468.

Radak, Z., Taylor, A. W., Sasvari, M., Ohno, H., Horkay, B., Furesz, J., Gaal, D. Telomerase activity is not altered by regular strenuous exercise in skeletal muscle or by sarcoma in liver of rats. *Redox Report*, 6:99-03.

Radak, Z., Gaal, D., Taylor, A. W., Kaneko, T., Tahara, S., Nakamoto, H., Goto, H. (2001). Attenuation of the development of murine solid leukemia tumor by physical exercise. *Antioxid. Redox Signal, 2002*, 4:213-219.

Rammazini B. (1700). *Diseases of Workers* (Latin). Translated by Wright. New York: Hafner, 1964 and by B. Delin, G. Gerhardson, and P. Nelson. Karlskrona: Abrahamsons, 1991 pp. 138-139.

Reddy B. S., Sugie S., Lowenfels A. (1988). Effect of voluntary exercise on azoxymethane-induced colon carcinogenesis in male F344 rats. *Cancer Research* Dec15 48(24Pt1):7079-81.

Rockhill, B., Willett, V. C., Hunter, D. J., Hankinson, S. E., Spiegelman, D., Colditz, G. A. (1998). Physical activity and breast cancer in a cohort of young women. *J-Natl-Cancer-Inst* Aug5 Vol. 90(15), pp. 1155-60.

Rodin, S. N. and Rodin, A. S. (2000). Human lung cancer and p53: The interplay between mutagenesis and selection. *Proceedings of the National Academy of Sciences of the USA*, Vol. 97., pp. 12 244-12 249.

Roebuck B. D., McCaffrey J., Baumgartner K. J. (1990). Protective effect of voluntary exercise during the postinitiation phase of pancreatic carcinogenesis in the rat. *Cancer Research* Nov1 Vol. 50(21), pp. 6811-6.

Severson, R. K., Nomura, A. M., Grove, J. S., and Stemmmeman, G. N. (1989). A prospective analysis of physical activity and cancer. *American Journal of Epidemiology* Vol. 130., pp. 522-529.

Shephard, R. J., and Futcher, R. (1997). Physical activity and cancer: how may protection be maximized? *Crit Rev Oncology*, Vol. 8., pp. 219-272.

Slattery, M. L., Schumacher, M. C., Smith, K. R., West, D. W., and Abd-Efghany, N. (1988). Physical activity, diet, and risk of colon cancer in Utah. *American Journal of Epidemiology*. Vol. 128., pp. 989-999.

Slattery, M. L., Potter, J. D., Curtin, K., Edwrads, S., Ma, K. N., Anderson, K., Schaffer, D., Samowitz, W. S. (2001). Estrogens reduce and withdrawal of esrtogens increase risk of microsatellite instability-positive colon cancer. *Cancer Research* Jan1 Vol. 61(1), pp. 126-30.

Smith, G. D., Shipley, M. J., Batty, G. D., Morris, J. N., and Marmot, M. (2000). Physical activity and cause-specific mortality in the Whitehall study. *American Journal of Public Health*, Vol. 114., pp. 1-8.

Steenland, K., Nowlin, S., and Palu, S. (1995). Cancer incidence in the National Health and Nutrition Survey 1. Follow-up data: diabetes, cholesterol, pulse, and physical activity. *Cancer Epidemiol. Biomarkers Prev.*, Vol. 4., pp. 807-811.

Suggie, S., Reddy, B. S., Lowenfels, A., Tanaka, T., Mori, H. (1992). Effect of voluntary exercise on azyzomethane-induced hepatocarcinogenesis in male F344 rats. *Cancer Letters* Mar31 Vol. 63(1), pp. 67-72.

Suzuki K., Machida K., Kariya M. (1992). (Conditoins for low-intensity voluntary wheel running in rats and its chronic effects on health indexes) *Nippon Eiseigaku Zasshi. Japanese* Dec Vol. 47(5), pp. 939-51.

Szent-Gyorgyi A. (1968). Bioelectronics. Intermolecular electron transfer may play a major role in biological regulation, defense, and cancer. *Science* 161:988-90

Swerdlow, J. A. and Green, A. (1987). Melanocytic naevi and melanoma: an epidemiological perspective. *British Journal of Dermatology*, Vol. 117., pp. 137-146.

Tang, R., Wang, J. Y., Lo, S. K., Hsieh, L. L. (1999). Physical activity, water intake and risk of colorectal cancer in Taiwan, a hospital based case-control study. *International Journal of Cancer* Aug12 82(4):484-9.

Taparowsky, E., Suard, Y., Fasano, O., Shimizu, K., Goldfarb, M. and Wigler, M. (1982). Activation of the T24 bladder carcinoma transforming gene is linked to a single amino acid change. *Nature*, Vol 300., pp. 762-

Tavani, A., Braga, C., La Vecchia C., Conti, E., Filiberti, R., Montella, M., Amadori, D., Russo, A., Franceschi, S. (1999). Physical activity and risk of cancers of colon and rectum: an Italian care control study. *British Journal of Cancer* Apr Vol. 79(11-12), pp. 1912-6.

Taylor, H., Klepetar, E., Keys, A., Parlin, W., Blackburn, H., and Puchner, T. (1962). Death rates among physically active and sedentary employees of the railroad industry. *American Journal of Public Health*, Vol. 52., pp. 1697-1707.

Taylor, R. S., Ramirez, R. D., Ogoshi, M., Chaffins, M., Piatyszek, M. A., and Shay, J.W. (1996). Detection of telomerase activity in malignant and nonmalignant skin conditions. *Journal of Investigative Dermatology*, Vol. 106., pp. 759-765.

Thompson H. (1994). Effect of exercise intensity and duration on the induction of mammary carcinogenesis. *Cancer Research*, Vol. 54., pp. 1960-1963.

Thompson, H. J., Westerlind, K. C., Snedden, J., Briggs, S., Singh, M. (1995). Exercise intensity dependent inhibition of 1-methyl-1-nitrosourea induced mammary carcinogenesis in female F-344 rats. *Carcinogenesis*, Aug Vol. 16(8), pp. 17836.

Thompson, H.J., Westerlind, K.C., Snedden, J., Briggs, S. and Singh, M. (1995). Exercise intensity dependent inhibition of methyl-1-nitrosourea induced mammary carcinogenesis in female F-344 rats. *Carcinogenesis*, Vol. 16., pp. 1783-1786.

Thorling, E. B. (1999). The effect of treadmill exercise on azozymethane-induced intestinal neoplasia in the male Fischer rat on two different high fat diets. *Nurt-Cancer*, Vol. 22(1),pp. 31-41.

Thune, I. and Lund, E. (1997). The influence of physical activity on lung-cancer risk: a prospective study of 81,516 men and women. *International Journal of Cancer*, Vol. 70., pp. 57-62.

Thune, I., Brenn, T., Lund, E., Gaard, M. (1997). Physical activity and the risk of breast cancer. *New England Journal of Medicine*, May Vol. 336(18), pp. 1269-75.

Tierney, L. M., McPhee, S.J., Papadakis, M. A. (Edited by) (1996). Current Medical Diagnosis & Tratment. Appleton & Lange, Stamford, CT.

Trentin, L., Ballon, G., Ometto, L., Perin, A., Basso, U., Chieco-Bianchi, L., Semenzato, G. and de Rossi, A. (1999). Telomerase activity in chronic lymphoproliferative disorders of B-cell lineage. *British Journal of Haematology*, Vol. 106, pp. 662-668.

Vena, J. E., Graham, S., Zielezny, M., Swanson, M. K., Barnes, R. E. & Nolan, J. (1985). Lifetime occupational exercise and colon cancer. *American Journal of Epidemiology*, Vol. 122.,pp. 357-365.

Wannamethee, G., Shaper, A. G., Macfarlane, P. W. (1993). Heart rate, physical activity and mortality from cancer and other noncardiovscular diseases. *American Journal of Epidemiology*, Vol. 137., pp. 735-748.

Weng, N., Levine, B. L., June, C.H. and Hodes, R. J. (1996). Regulated expression of telomerase activity in human T lymphocyte development and activation. *Journal of Experimental Medicine*, Vol. 183, pp. 2471-2479.

Whitaker, N. J., Bryan, T. M., Bonnefin, P., Chang, A. C-M., Musgrove, E. A., Braithwaite, A.W. and Reddel, R.R. (1995).Involvment of RB-1, p53, p16[INK4] and telomerase in immortalisation of human cells. *Oncogene*, Vol. 11., pp. 971-976.

White, E., Jacobs, E. J., Daling, J. R. (1996). Physical activity in relation to colon cancer in middle-aged men and women. *American Journal of Epidemiology* Jul, Vol. 144(1), pp. 42-50.

Whittal, K. S., Parkhouse, W. S. (1996). Exercise during adolescence and its effects mammary gland development, proliferation, and nytrosomethylemia (NMU) induced tumorigenesis is rats. *Breast Cancer Research and Treatment*, Vol. 37(1), pp. 21-7.

Whittal-Strange K. S., Chadan, S., Parkhouse, W. S., Chadau, S. (1998). Exercise during puberty and NMU-induced mammary tumorigenesis in rats. *Breast Cancer Research and Treatment* Jan, Vol. 47(1), pp.1-8.

Yasumoto, S., Kunimura, C., Kikuchi, K., Tahara, H., Ohiji, H., Yamamoto, H., Ide, T. and Utakoji, T. (1996). Telomerase activity in normal human epithelial cells. *Oncogene*, Vol. 13., pp. 433-439.

Yeo, C. J. (1999). Tumor suppressor genes: A short review. *Surgery*, Vol. 125., pp. 363-366.

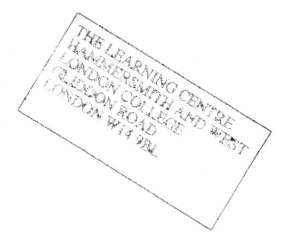